THE CULTURE OF
ADOLESCENT RISK-TAKING

CULTURE AND HUMAN DEVELOPMENT
A Guilford Series

Sara Harkness
Charles M. Super
Editors

THE CULTURE OF ADOLESCENT RISK-TAKING
Cynthia Lightfoot

PLAYING ON THE MOTHER-GROUND:
CULTURAL ROUTINES FOR CHILDREN'S DEVELOPMENT
David F. Lancy

JAPANESE CHILDREARING:
TWO GENERATIONS OF SCHOLARSHIP
David W. Shwalb and Barbara J. Shwalb, Editors

PARENTS' CULTURAL BELIEF SYSTEMS:
THEIR ORIGINS, EXPRESSIONS, AND CONSEQUENCES
Sara Harkness and Charles M. Super, Editors

CULTURE AND ATTACHMENT:
PERCEPTIONS OF THE CHILD IN CONTEXT
Robin L. Harwood, Joan G. Miller, and Nydia Lucca Irizarry

SIBLINGS IN SOUTH ASIA:
BROTHERS AND SISTERS IN CULTURAL CONTEXT
Charles W. Nuckolls, Editor

The Culture of Adolescent Risk-Taking

Cynthia Lightfoot

FOREWORD BY JAAN VALSINER

THE GUILFORD PRESS
New York   London

© 1997 The Guilford Press
A Division of Guilford Publications, Inc.
72 Spring Street, New York, NY 10012

Printed in the United States of America

This book is printed on acid-free paper.

Last digit is print number: 9 8 7 6 5 4 3 2 1

Library of Congress Cataloging-in-Publication Data

Lightfoot, Cynthia.
    The culture of adolescent risk-taking / Cynthia Lightfoot;
foreword by Jaan Valsiner.
       p.   cm.—(Culture and human development)
    Includes bibliographical references and index.
    ISBN 1-57230-189-9 (hard).—ISBN 1-57230-232-1 (pbk.)
    1. Adolescence.   2. Risk-taking (Psychology) in adolescence.
I. Series.
HQ796.L444   1997
305.235—dc21   96-47250
                                     CIP

To my teachers

Acknowledgments

I would like to express my deeply felt appreciation to everyone—family, friends, colleagues—who helped me with this project. I am especially grateful to the Series Editors, Sara Harkness and Charles Super, for this opportunity, and the generosity of their time and encouragement; to Jaan Valsiner, for his friendship and good counsel; and to the teenagers who shared with me their thoughts and stories.

CYNTHIA LIGHTFOOT

Foreword
Interpretive Adventures in the World of the Adolescent

This little book constitutes a milestone in a number of ways. Aside from being a great adventure for its author to integrate her various interests, which have survived all the social pressures inherent in academic life, the book has a place in the vastly growing chorus of efforts to study adolescence. Yet psychologists are rarely reflective about what they mean by "study." Usually, what is implied is the need to get more data about how adolescents differ from adults—adolescents usually being considered more "troublesome," "promiscuous," "idealistic," or whatever, than the perfectly "normal" adults (of whom the researcher considers him- or herself a most important representative).

It is in the arena of revealing adult mental and emotional blinders that this book makes its contribution. *Adolescence has been studied mostly from the vantage point of adults, and not from that of adolescents themselves.* The result of this is a selectivity in the research themes that are addressed, and the ways in which these themes are worked out. Once, when perusing an introductory child psychology textbook published in the United States, I came to understand just how limiting these blinders can be. What struck me was the adamantly negative tone with which the textbook authors provided empirical evidence about the ages at which children begin to have sexual encounters. When viewed in the context of the history of U.S. society in this century, this age seems to move downwards. The textbook on that subject read almost like a sensationalistic newspaper report, revealing the horrors of sinfulness creeping into the innocent lives of U.S. middle-class family environments, at an increasingly early age. What was completely absent was any coverage of the adolescents' own personal interpretations of their first (or later) sexual encounters.

This example seemed to me more than curious. If the psychology of adolescence (as a subpart of child psychology) is to be knowledgeable about the psychological phenomena of adolescence (in contrast to relying on adult gossip about teenagers, enhanced by journalistic reports), then it is adolescents' personal feelings and thoughts about these sexual encounters that psychologists should be studying (and reporting in textbooks, which are oriented toward postadolescents). Yet that facet of study is mostly absent, and a curious blend of sociological or epidemiological data mixed with the ideology of a sociomoral culture replaces psychological investigation. After learning the titillating fact that children enter into sexual relations earlier now than some decades ago, we have not learned anything about their *psychological* development. We have merely added another "Trivial Pursuit" kind of fact to our discourse, failing to interpret it in terms of psychological analysis. It may be good fodder for adults' laments about the "difficulties" of living with adolescents, and how infinitely "worried" they as parents are about any possible "wrongdoings" by their precious children—yet the value of such uninterpreted facts for general science is minimal.

In general, research on adolescents in contemporary psychology proceeds with ideologically preordained scenarios for how one or another topic is to be studied. Thus, early entrance into sexual encounters, or trying drugs, writing graffiti, beating up next-neighborhood gangs, and skipping school are to be studied as part of the category of *problems* of adolescence (i.e., problems for the age cohort of their parents, to whom psychologists also tend to belong). Adolescents are often viewed as being "at risk" for almost anything—except for being considered "problematic" by their own parents or teachers. And, certainly, adolescents do not easily let adult investigators enter their personal worlds, veiling the latter in secrecy, peer group maintenance of shared meanings, and pure arrogance toward "adults trying to tell me how I should be again."

The author of this book should be complimented for her careful work in overcoming the divide that usually separates adult researchers and adolescent research participants. In order to accomplish this, she has had to disappoint many a parent, who might have considered their signature on the "parental consent form" to be a foot in the door toward entering into the personal world of their own home-grown "foreigner"—their adolescent son or daughter. Parental control over their adolescents with the help of the researcher, and research results, was not permitted. Although parents may have been disappointed with the research, adolescents themselves were not. The result is a glimpse into the world of adolescents with the help of these very adolescents, who were actually eager to teach the author about things that fascinated, bothered, or merely bored them in their lives. The result is that almost all of the topics that appear to be "problems" or "risk factors," from the perspective of adults, constitute a realm of personal construction of meaningful events for adolescents. These events may be transitory, episodic, knowingly antisocietal, yet their thrilling and adventuresome nature is created and interpreted by adolescents, just as the adults attribute negative significance to such episodes, and often try to limit them from happening through strict rules and disciplinary practices.

In studying the personal culture of adolescents, psychologists' knowledge base can only advance by looking through the eyes of adolescents, who make their own meetings of life events. Large-scale epidemiological studies of this population, with no individual depth of analysis of the personal phenomena, are unlikely to lead us to new understanding. In contrast, careful study of individual cases in terms of their systemic organization can lead to novelty.

However, it is not an easy task in present-day North American psychology to get to the "voices of adolescence" and let those be central in the empirical data. In this historical time of a society dominated by the business of law, with mass media readily making scapegoats out of anybody, research with human subjects has become increasingly censored by social institutions, and self-censored by investigators. Topics that are not welcome in social interaction in the given society—sex, religion, salaries, and so forth—are easy targets for censorship by institutional academic review boards (or "ethics committees," as these are often labeled). A curious difference between the social roles of psychologists and journalists emerges:

Researchers in psychology are censored as to what questions they are allowed to ask their participants for research purposes (with anything "too sensitive" being changed or suppressed), whereas at the same time journalists may create their own "symbolic capital" by asking the very same questions (and more dramatic, if not traumatic ones) with a full view of the interviewed person appearing on television. Psychologists, bowing to the stance of institutional review boards, explain their avoidance of "sensitive topics" by reference to the "protection of the subjects." Somehow, these concerns seem not to apply to interviews on similar topics in the area of mass media.

Emphasizing the issue of the social regulation of psychologists' research activities can easily be interpreted as "politically incorrect"—and in this land of increased emphasis on self-censorship of language use, or on "political correctness," that would be a rather sinful act. Yet it is a serious issue for science: "Political correctness" as a starting point for a scientific psychology of adolescence would guarantee a result that serves the purposes of the social institutions of the adults, and stigmatizes or pathologizes adolescents. Such science would be an example of "colonial science"—adolescents here would be similar to the indigenous populations of colonized lands, with researchers studying them from the viewpoint of the colonizers (adults). Elimination of the rights of adolescents—if we speak in terms of moral or legal discourse—would emerge from such research. Paradoxically, by guiding psychologists away from asking "sensitive" questions of research participants, the latter are not "protected," but exploited, for these aspects of the researched phenomena do not trouble the researchers, thus maintaining the institutionally constructed interpretive orientations.

An interesting scenario is to imagine what research questions *adolescent* researchers would ask of their *adult* "research participants," if the roles were reversed. Evidence for these topics emerges from the materials in this book. Perhaps one topic could be the relationship of parents' interpretation of adolescence as a "risk factor" to parents' distrustfulness and need for control of the adolescents? And I expect that adolescent researchers would want to measure their parents' authoritarianism along the lines of Theodor Adorno's elaboration of the "fascist personality" type in the post-World War II period.

Even if this reversal is a game about what topics might be important, the point is simple—the encounters with adults that are found problematic by adolescents would be suggested for research. The result would be scientifically substantiated stigmatization of the adults (by adolescents), in ways that the powerful social group (in this reversal game—adolescents) protects by way of insistence on "political correctness." Last, but not least, the world has already experienced at least one such role reversal (though not in the area of research)—the period of "cultural revolution" in China reversed the meanings of "political correctness" in the parent–adolescent relationship. The potential power of the united efforts of adolescents has been recognized by politicians, and has been used both for ruling through "divide and govern" tactics, and for occasional political purposes.

This possible reversibility of perspectives brings the question of science as interpretive practice to the center of attention. If psychological research on adolescence is preoriented by socioinstitutional ideologies—and there are a number of those—then the orientation of such perspectives is indeed a "hermeneutic" task. The complexity of the different "voices" in this process is not only on the researcher's side. Similar complexity occurs in the case of the researched: A girl who puts on her makeup in her room, then rushes by her parents to enjoy the thrill of their horror, and escapes to be picked up by friends before the parents come to their senses and try to "control" the girl, is involved in a complex dialogue within herself, not to speak of the obvious one with parents. *Complexity of the dialogical processes in adolescence has not been matched with methods on the side of researchers that adequately represent that complexity in the empirical evidence.* The efforts that readers see in this book are but a small step in this direction, still far from where the discipline needs to be. Just relabeling science into an "interpretive" role does not clarify how that interpretation takes place. It merely states that it is the meaning-making that is the center of focus, yet it can occur in many ways.

All in all, the present book is an invitation to enter into the world of psychological phenomena as an adventure that adults have rarely allowed themselves since the time of their own adolescence, or at least since the last time the reader enjoyed reading *Huckleberry Finn*. As an invitation to such adventure, this book provides thrilling moments, which, after all, science should create. The author demonstrates that the psychology of adolescence need be neither trivial nor "correct." Instead, the adolescents who see their curious world in very personal ways can tell us something about ourselves that we may not have tried to discover since passing through that period of "storm and stress" ourselves, largely forgetting it. Refreshing our memories in innovative ways is a worthwhile result of a peek into the culture of the adolescents.

JAAN VALSINER
Brasilia, D.F., July 1996

Contents

THE CULTURE OF
ADOLESCENT RISK-TAKING

CHAPTER 1

Introduction

PRELUDE

For this book I tried to harness together a few ideas from different disciplines, mainly anthropology and psychology, and drive them toward an understanding of the culture of adolescent risk-taking. My aim is to communicate a reasonably coherent perspective on culture, adolescents, and risk-taking, which has emerged by fits and starts over the course of several years. During this time I read widely—of adolescents and risk-taking, naturally—but also of play, drama, narrative, and aesthetics, and how these categories of action and experience contribute to the development of self and culture. This is because I went into the project with the idea that adolescent risk-taking has much in common with these other forms of action. Consider its play-like aspects: It often conveys a "don't have to" or a "just for the hell of it" attitude, and, like play, it can provide commentary about the players and how they understand and interpret each other and the larger scheme of things. Risks may express, for example, a thumb-to-nose defiance of authority. They can convey one's commitment to a group of peers. They can speak to the history of one's relationship with a specific individual (some risks can be taken with acquaintances, whereas others are shared only with close friends). In all of these cases, or from all of these interpretive levels of analysis, risk-taking is a way of framing the world—certain significant portions of it, anyway.

Risk-taking can also be considered in terms of its dramatic structure and aesthetic properties: It is imaginative, inventive, uncertain, and goes beyond the ordinary and predictable in ways that can titillate, excite, and very often frighten. It has an emotional current.

In contrast to the passing and passive flow of "mere experience," taking a risk is to seek or to have "*an* experience," and as Victor Turner suggests, *an* experience, "like a rock in a Zen sand garden, stands out from the evenness of passing hours and years and forms what Dilthey called a 'structure of experience.' In other words, it does not have an *arbitrary* beginning and ending, cut out of the stream of chronological temporality, but has what Dewey called 'an initiation and a consummation'" (Turner, 1986, p. 35; original italics).

Turner goes on to argue that it is in structured experience, or "processual units of experience" (p. 38) that we find meaning, the deepest sort of which is aesthetic. I will make a case for construing adolescents' risks in similar terms, as structured, "cultural experience," as protoaesthetic forms. We will examine the extent to which risks are actively sought for their capacity to challenge, excite, and transform oneself and one's relationships with others. In this regard, risks are speculative, experimental, and oriented toward some uncertain and wished-for future.

And if risk-taking can be said to begin as play and drama, then it ends as narrative and story. There has been a ground swell of recent interest in the role of *narrative* in self-development—narrative as both process and product, that is, as meaning-construction and story (e.g., Bruner, 1986; Gergen & Gergen, 1983; Hankiss, 1981; Peacock & Holland, 1993; Rosaldo, 1986; Sarbin, 1986). The thrust of this work is that people weave life experiences into coherent stories, or narratives, in ways that reconstruct images of themselves and the groups or communities with which they affiliate. Narrative and storytelling is considered integral to identity formation, and is thought to play an important role in constructing a sense of personal and cultural continuity: It provides an avenue for establishing connectedness and coherence across human actions and life events, and permits a sense of movement through time (Crites, 1986; Hallowell, 1955; Howard, 1985). Theodore Sarbin, an early proponent of narrative psychology, went so far as to argue that *narrative* be embraced as a root metaphor in psychology (1986). His "narratory principle" is that "human beings think, perceive, imagine, and make moral choices according to narrative structures" (p. 8).

Teenagers tell and retell their adventures, and this is significant action, both socially and personally. Like the hunting, fishing, and war stories analyzed by anthropologists, adolescents' risks can be seen to promote a sense of shared history, and a means by which to mediate ingroup–outgroup relations. Risks provide material for stories. They become part of the collective biography of group experience. Magnified by the symbolic meanings of the group, they can, and sometimes do, assume nearly mythical proportions.

RECRUITING AND INTERVIEWING THE TEENAGERS

In addition to the theoretical work, much time was taken poring over transcripts of discussions with adolescents who were asked about risk-taking, about what it means to be a teenager, and about their own personal risk involvement. Because one of the major aims of this endeavor was to explore the culture of risk-taking, it was important to locate individuals within a nexus of social life. I was interested in identifying groups of adolescents who hung out together, and in all likelihood, took risks together, so a cluster sampling procedure was used to recruit participants. I began with one teenager that I knew personally (I was friendly with his mother, actually). I called him, outlined the project, and asked if he would be interested in participating. He agreed to an interview. Afterwards, I asked for names and numbers of friends he thought might also be interested. These individuals were interviewed, asked for names of possibly interested friends, and so forth. In this way, I worked through a network of 41 teenagers who were more or less closely associated with one another.

The initial contact with participants and their parents was by telephone. The teenager was contacted first, informed of the purpose and procedures of the study, and asked if he or she would be interested in talking with me. Only two declined, saying that they were "too busy." The others were surprisingly enthusiastic. I had expected recruitment to be a long and arduous process, complicated by lack of interest, missed appointments, and so forth. But this was far from the case. A few of the teenagers acted as liaisons between myself and other interested teens. My name and telephone number were given out, and several individuals contacted me, asking for interviews. On a few occasions, individuals showed up for interviews with friends in tow. Appointments were made on the spot.

I am still not clear on what accounted for this eagerness. Perhaps adolescents simply enjoy talking about themselves and the risks they take. More likely, I think, is their desire to do things together, especially things that are out of the ordinary, be it taking risks, trying out for sports, dropping out of school, or participating in a research project.

After getting permission from the teenager, it was explained that parental consent would be required, and arrangements were make to speak with a parent or guardian. Only one declined, again on the grounds that the child was "too busy." Most of the others, after hearing my synopsis of the project, expressed interest and amusement. "Risk-taking? Yeah, you've called the right number," or, "He's grounded right now, but if you want to talk to him next week that would be fine." Although ready to work around the vastly complicated school, sport, and social lives of the teenagers, I was taken aback by the extent to which their risk-taking (or, more properly, its consequences) became a scheduling issue. One teenager had to reschedule an appointment because his jaw had been wired shut. After the swelling subsided, I heard through unnaturally clenched teeth that in an altered state of reason, and a failed imitation of Tarzan, he had splayed his face on the trunk of a tree.

Beyond their general amusement, the parents were very much interested in the project. Based on my assumptions about the type of person inclined to read through a book of this sort, it is within reason to say that the teenagers interviewed and described in these pages are very much like your own, or the ones next door. The fact that I drew largely from a population of middle- and upper-middle-class professional families was never more apparent than in the questions posed by the parents. One asked if I would be using a random sample or a stratified random sample. When I told her that I was interested in interviewing teenagers who knew one another, she expressed concern about the generality of the results. Most were relatively good-natured about their teenagers' risk involvement and considered it a phase that all would survive, God willing. Nevertheless, they were often incredulous at the inconstancy of their children's reasoning. I was told of children who were mathematically brilliant, politically savvy, artistically gifted, yet totally irrational, foolish, and uncommunicative about their social lives. Still, risk-taking was considered part of what it means to be a teenager, in much the same way that learning to walk is part of being a toddler. One father, in fact, worried that he son didn't take *enough* risks. "I don't know," he mused, "he has a lot of friends and he's real active in sports, but he just doesn't take many risks. It worries me sometimes—I think kids learn a lot from it." Issues of confidentiality prevented me from calling him later to assuage his anxiety.

By the time all was said and done, I had interviewed 41 teenagers, 22 boys and 19 girls. All were between the ages of 16 and 18 years. Because they were all associated with one another to a greater or lesser extent by virtue of the sampling method, they were also fairly homogeneous demographically. They lived in a fairly typical university town: an affluent community located in the Raleigh–Durham–Chapel Hill area of North Carolina. The racial constitution was predominantly white, with the exception of one black and one Asian American. Almost all attended the same public high school serving a middle- and upper-middle-class neighborhood; one attended a Quaker Friends School, and two were high school dropouts. Within this network of 41, five discrete groups were discernible, that is, five groups of teenagers who did most of their risk-taking with one another. The methods for determining these groups will be described later. For now, it is perhaps best to think of them in terms of Dunphy's concept of small, intimate cliques more or less integrated within a larger crowd.

Each teenager was interviewed twice, in a location of his or her choice. Typically, the first interview was conducted in the teenager's home. This had the advantage of meeting the individual on terra firma, and also of meeting a parent, usually the mother. The main objective of this interview was to establish rapport, and it focused primarily on driving experiences. Most of the teenagers had recently received their driver's licenses, were excited about driving, and enthusiastic about discussing their experiences and risks taken behind the wheel. At the conclusion of this interview, which lasted about an hour, arrangements were made for a second meeting. For this, I said, "We can meet here, again, or anywhere else you like." Virtually all chose a different location, several commenting on the advantages of a more private setting. "Private," as it turned out, meant "away from parents" and, preferably, all others like them. So the second interview was usually conducted in a local teenage "hangout." Hangouts included parks, shopping malls, fast food restaurants, libraries, and coffee shops—all sufficiently public to ensure the privacy of a conversation. The second interview lasted approximately 2 hours. The teenagers were asked questions meant to assess their understanding of risk, and completed a checklist in which they indicated their preferences for exciting or novel experiences in different interpersonal circumstances (e.g., getting to know someone of the same or opposite sex). They were also read and questioned about different scenarios in which adolescent story characters were portrayed as engaging in specific risks. Finally, they were asked to reflect on their own risk experiences—what they did, with whom, and why.

In these semistructured interviews, the teenagers also discussed boyfriends and girlfriends, parents, future plans, jobs, and a variety of other topics. Some were relevant to their risk involvement, others entirely beside the point. Regarding the former, I did my best to encourage the expression of individual differences in the importance attached to any particular topic. For example, some individuals perceived family relationships as having a major influence on their risks. This was particularly true for those who considered their parents either excessively overbearing or lackadaisical. For others, however, family relationships seemed less relevant, or only quietly relevant, as I will discuss later. General rapport was another consideration. I had invited the teenagers to report experiences that they typically shield from adult eyes. This agenda, and good manners, dictated that I do my best to make them feel comfortable and in control of the situation.

There was also considerable variation in the types of risks reported. They ranged from those that would make any parent proud, to those that would embarrass, or terrify. I was told of intellectual and physical challenges—trying out for the Math Club, or mountain climbing, for example; of risks related to dating and interpersonal relationships; of pranks both clever and mean spirited; of mixing drugs and alcohol with sex, with driving, with each other. The risks varied in meaning, intention, and consequence. They were linked, often simultaneously, to rebelliousness and authority structures; to peer process and interpersonal desire; to feelings of esteem, confidence, maturity. Meaning layered on meaning, intention on intention, consequence on consequence, risk on risk: they were polysemous and open to multiple interpretations, as expressed in the following detailed and articulate account of why risk-taking is appealing to teenagers:

> "I don't want to say we feel invincible, because we don't; we're very aware that we can die. But by the same token, we're in the prime of our life and we have excellent health. We take more risks because we're getting independence. Also because there's so much pressure—at school and to meet your parents' demands and everything. It's generally fun because you're putting your life on the line. Once again, it's not that we feel invincible. It's that release. This is my personal feeling even though medically it may be wrong: Besides the psychological aspects, there are real physical, emotional outlets such as the release of adrenaline, like when you laugh chemicals are released in your brain which reduce stress and things like that. And mental, like I said, taking risks, having fun, basically [relieving] stress. And there are other things. Even though people deny it and I deny it, sometimes to spite your parents, even though you're usually just hurting yourself. Risk puts your life or your trust and status at risk. A nonrisk doesn't challenge you, doesn't put anything in jeopardy. Everything is a risk—risk and challenge. Otherwise you just go insane."

That risks, and the propensity to take them, can be multiply determined should not be taken to mean, however, that a given risk provides a blank page upon which an interested party may inscribe *any* interpretation, or that multiple interpretations appear in the manner of a palimpsest of partial, obscure, or conflicting texts. More often than not, the multiplicity of interpretations adhered to was constrained by different structured, relational levels, which varied from the most general cultural and historical, to the most subjective and psychological. Thus, at one level we have the teenager's social position as an adolescent in contemporary American society. Other levels include his or her position and relationships with family, with peers, and, finally, with him- or herself—this last relationship having to do with the expectations, desires, and goals embraced as relevant to self-definition and -development. The preeminent task, then, was to try to get a handle on the processes through which risks come to carry and provoke certain meanings and interpretations at these different relational levels, and the significance of this meaning-making for adolescents' development.

GENERAL THEMES

My efforts to understand adolescent risk-taking as play, structured experience, and narrative led me toward a certain theoretical orientation that has become increasingly ascendant in philosophy, history, and literary theory, as well as the social sciences. The "interpretive perspective," as it will be known here, is meant to locate the actions of persons within the symbolic forms, communicative practices, and shared idioms of culture. This makes it especially well suited to focusing my interests in adolescent development and cultural experience. From this perspective, risk-taking is taken as meaningful action. As such, it can be understood as a form of experience that is shared between individuals who know and act toward one another on the basis of particular points of view, which are constructed, articulated, and clarified over time and in the course of social participation. Taking a risk narrates and dramatizes point of view, and sharing a risk is a statement of likemindedness, of common purpose or perspective. By these lights it can be seen as an expressive form, a social drama that organizes action and experience, and contributes to definitions of self.

Several themes are developed, all of which will be seen to hover around the matter of characterizing the relationship between persons and culture, a task made all the more interesting, and difficult, by the need to navigate through those several levels at which the relationship is manifested. Thus, for example, much will be made of the relationship between the developing adolescent and adolescent peer culture, often borrowing ideas and analyses developed by psychologists, anthropologists, sociologists, and folklorists who examine the culture of younger children. There is, in fact, a burgeoning and illuminating literature, much of it reviewed in Chapter 4, that takes the cultural artifacts and folklore of preschool- and school-age children, and explores the processes through which they clarify and communicate a sense of self and social identity. During adolescence, however, the artifacts of childhood are thrown over for those that are better suited to newly arriving concerns of the self. So it is that the whole hop, skip, and jump of children's culture—the scripts of their fantasy play, their school yard games, bathroom humor, stories, slang—become pieces of a distant life more fitted to a scrapbook than to the identity-seeking needs of the adolescent.

Adolescents are makers of new talismans. The clothes they wear, their music and media choices, their language and slang, their hangouts: all of these are forms expressing who they are, and who they would like to be. Borrowing a term from Donald Winnicott (1971), these talismans are the "transitional objects" of adolescence, and I will argue that risk-taking be included among them. Transitional objects, or transitional spaces, are playful, speculative, and imaginative rapprochements of fact and fantasy. The character of the transitional space is redefined throughout the lifecourse, from the play of young children, to the "cultural experience" (scientific and aesthetic) of adults; but its transitional nature—the osmosis of what is and what might be—is invariant, and on that score Winnicott claimed an identity between such apparently disparate phenomenon as seeing a horse in a broomstick and entertaining a scientific hypothesis (Lightfoot, in press-a). Both are imaginative constructions that structure and give meaning to future action. They are a means of apprehending reality, and in that way define a leading edge to the organization of experience. So, too, adolescent risk-taking. Like popular media preferences, political attitudes, and clothing choices, risks have a significant role to play in organizing action and experience, and in structuring a sense of self and social identity. Risks and reputations are mutually affirming. Rednecks, I was told, drink beer, smoke pot, and like to fight. Preps, on the other hand, smoke cigarettes, snort coke, and drive fast cars. Certain risks, or patterns of risks, are symbolic of certain kinds of social identity. Worn like badges—of autonomy, or defiance, or group membership—risks are declarations of the self.

My interest thus extends beyond the specific material or behavioral artifacts of adolescent culture. I am concerned more particularly with the developmental and interpretive processes by which "objects" become artifactual, symbolic, or semiotic. Construed as interpretive process, adolescents' risks tell us something not only about how teenagers understand risk types and group types (or "crowd" types), but how they understand themselves in relation to their friends, in relation to their parents and teachers, and also in relation to culture in the broadest sense. In their reflections on risk-taking and interpersonal relations, for example, adolescents described shared risks as promoting cohesion, trust, and closeness. Risks were understood as vehicles for initiating new relationships or group memberships, and consolidating or maintaining existing relationships. It was also the consensus that, as adolescents, they were *expected* to take risks. One participant referred to risk-taking as "the natural code of teenagers." Indeed, a lot of the teenagers confirmed that much of their risk activity occurs only in the presence of other teens:

> "It seems like the laws in this country are arranged so that you can't have any fun without taking a risk. It is so boring to drive the speed limit and it seems like people accept you more if you're, like, a dangerous driver or something. If there is a line of cars going down the road and the other lane is clear and you pass eight cars at once, everybody likes that. I passed eight cars yesterday. Seeing everybody see you do that, like, if you pass eight of your friends cars. . . . If my friends are with me in the car, or if there are a lot of people in the line, I would do it, but if I'm by myself and I didn't know anybody then I wouldn't do it. That's no fun."

In addition to their interpersonal significance, risks are relevant to intergroup dynamics. For example, the analysis of specific groups of risk-takers showed that risk involvement is associated with group integration into the larger teen culture. Some risks are normative within the larger community. In this one, just about everyone drank alcohol, went to parties, and maybe smoked a bit of pot. This is all part of a larger teen culture, and individuals engaged in these normative risks had frequent contact with others outside their primary clique. Other risks, however, were considered more deviant (frequent and heavy drug use, in this group of teenagers), and isolated those involved from the larger community, and thus, potential sources of growth and new patterns of action.

In the same way that risks can be understood to comment on peers and peer culture, they reveal connections to parents and other authorities. The interview material indicates that risks stand as declarations of independence and autonomy, as acts of rebellion against an authority imposed by others. It is a private rebellion, however, because the aim is never to bare one's anger or disaffection with authority openly but rather to avoid the direct confrontation that comes of getting caught. Sometimes the motive for avoiding confrontation is to maintain privileges—use of the car, going out, later curfew, and so forth. But many teenagers were genuinely concerned with maintaining the trust and respect of adults, especially their parents, and took care to avoid looking like "just another asshole teenager running around." One commented:

> "If I thought that what I was going to do was going to completely ruin their [parents'] whole concept of me then I wouldn't do it. I'm not going to do something that I think they're going to hate me for, even if I don't think they're going to find out about it. That's always been my big restriction."

Nevertheless, there is a clear sense of a developing autonomy: "We take more risks because we are breaking away from our parents and it is fun to test that freedom."

At the most abstract level, risk-taking may be interpreted in cultural–historical terms, and from this vantage point we will examine changing cultural conceptions of the role of experience in transforming lives. There is a certain and interesting ambivalence surrounding our views and attitudes toward risk-taking. We will find that risks and adventures are understood to entail a high potential for harm or loss, but are also acknowledged as demonstrations of character, or as sources of growth and opportunity. (Recall the father who worried that his son didn't take *enough* risks.) Hand in hand with this abiding ambivalence, however, are significant changes in how we understand the relationship between the risk and the risk-taker. We have developed, over the course of a few thousand years, a rather differentiated and integrated version of persons and their worlds. The current, modern view is that individuals are active seekers of experience who pursue novelty and risk for the explicit purpose of extending the horizons of their lives. But this has not always been the received view, in either science or literature. Literature and literary sources show that our modern conception—the current canon—emerged over the course of hundreds of years. We will spend a bit of time exploring, in particular, the evolution of novelistic forms, which culminates, finally, in the *Bildungsroman,* a form that focuses on the psychological development and education of the principal character. We will also look to the history of science and philosophy for evidence of the modern view and its incipient forms.

My purpose in developing the historical theme is twofold. First, because our cultural canonical forms are composed in present symbolic or semiotic practices, be they literary, philosophical, or scientific, they provide material for our own "world-making" or meaning-making (Bruner, 1986), for the way we go about the business of studying and interpreting our domain of interest. Because cultural forms are drawn into the framing of our action and understanding—as scholars, teachers, or parents of adolescents—they are integral to a generative process that results in new levels of understanding. In other words, knowing the cultural–historical dimensions of youth and adventure gives meaning and fresh insight into our contemporary views of adolescents and their behaviors. Second, because world-making is a principal function of mind (because, as Peirce, 1977, argues, matter is mind hidebound with habits) to understand the evolution of canonical forms is to gain insight into the ontogenesis of personal variants, of developing mind. Both are narrative achievements driven by the same interpretive processes. This is, of course, developmentalism writ large: In order to be scientists of human development, we need to be also historians of science and culture.

The keystone to all of this concerns the relationship between the personal and the canonical. It prods and pricks contemporary anthropological and psychological theories of self and cultural identity. It is a principal target for theories of play, narrative, semiotics, and aesthetics that explore the realm of the imaginative as an interstitial space between persons and cultural contexts. The imaginative realm, according to Winnicott (1971), is the "play space" we carve from everyday life. This is the location of cultural experience, where cultural forms are transformed as personal meanings. It is here that actions become meaningful and persons become themselves: This is the place where we live.

Taking a risk is to act within the imaginative sphere. It is speculation, experiment, and hypothesis. My point, in the end, is that the drama and daring of adolescent social life provides a vehicle for the imagination, which entrains culture in individuals, and contributes to the development and awareness of self as social participant. As play, drama, narrative, adolescent risk-taking is a means of framing and transforming mere experience as cultural experience. And taken in the spirit of Ortega's (1914/1961) observation that each adventure is a new birth of the world, how can it fail to be interesting?

CHAPTER 2

The History of Our Ambivalence

A teenager told me that "if you plod along and do the same boring old thing your whole damn life you'll die a boring old fart." This was to justify his risk involvement, which included sneaking out of the house in the middle of the night to share a joint with friends, skipping school to drop acid at the beach, and picking fights with rednecks and frat boys. My reaction was probably typical—good humor riding the tail of astonishment—and I suppose that the historical stamina of our interest in adolescent risk-taking owes some debt to the double meanings that we attach to these behaviors. On the one hand, many have gained notoriety as "social problems," manifestations of an insidious pathology overtaking the body of contemporary society. The sentiment is hardly overstated in a time during which teen violence and homicides roil suburbs and inner cities alike, and HIV moves rapidly and perniciously among the teen population. Yet we romanticize youth's disposition for mischief with equal enthusiasm. Our literature and folklore make heroes of young adventurers and invite nostalgic reflection on a time in our lives when taking risks created windows of possibility and was seen to test our mettle, if not our maturity. Throughout history we have brought these behaviors into focus with two apparently incompatible lenses. One provides a view of risk-taking as trouble, the other as opportunity.

RISK-TAKING AS TROUBLE: CHAUCER TO CONTEMPORARY THEORY

Popular interest in adolescents' risk involvement began even before the adults in their lives determined that they were coherent enough as a group to deserve a name, that is, before *adolescence* became a household word. G. Stanley Hall (1904) popularized this label for those between childhood and maturity, but its widespread acceptance had as much to do with larger social and economic processes as it did with the nature of teenagers themselves (see also Gillis, 1974; Kett, 1977; Schlegel & Barry, 1991). The most significant was the need for a formally educated citizenry created by the industrial revolution. As education for children became more systematized in the late 1800s and early 1900s, older children became more visible. We devised special school curricula for them, and beyond that, engineered social environments in which they spent large amounts of time hanging out with same-age peers. The adolescent peer group, in many ways an adaptation to these economic and educational reforms, came to supplant the mixed-age social groups of years past.

It is interesting, and telling, that at the time our society began to take note of adolescents and their groups, the eyes of educators, philosophers, and scientists turned quickly to their misbehaviors. Large boys, in particular, attracted much attention. They were widely recognized as being high-spirited, reckless, difficult to control, overconfident, and inclined to drop out of school (Kett, 1977). Teachers were called upon to address the special problems presented by those of their pupils who were in that awkward place between childhood and adulthood.

Still, we can reach back to a time before "adolescence" became embodied in school curricula, youth organizations, and judicial systems, that is, before it became institutionalized, and find references to individuals with a foot on each side of whatever it means to be fully mature. Even here they are replete with warnings of impending disaster. Plato proposed a minimum drinking age because "fire should not be poured upon fire"; Aristotle made much of youthful passions, impulses, and feelings of omniscience; Rousseau compared the adolescent to a lion in season, distrustful of his keeper and ungovernable.

> As the roaring of the waves precedes the tempest, so the murmur of rising passions announces this tumultuous change: a suppressed excitement warns us of the approaching danger. A change of temper, frequent outbreaks of anger, a perpetual stirring of the mind, make the child almost ungovernable. He becomes deaf to the voice he used to obey: he is a lion in a fever: he distrusts his keeper and refuses to be controlled. (Rousseau, 1762/1911, p. 175)

These vivid and often violent images of youth also color the pages of English literature from the Middle Ages to the present (Kiell, 1959; Violato & Wiley, 1990). Chaucer, Shakespeare, Milton, Wordsworth—all present a vision of youth as characteristically excessive, passionate, proud, and sensual, and contrast it with the clear-eyed sobriety of adulthood. Heightened affectivity is the primary culprit. It stands accused of inclining youth toward adventures in love and war (Chaucer's *Canterbury Tales*), and underlies the first classic tale of teen suicide (Shakespeare's *Romeo and Juliet*). It disrupts normal functioning, sometimes to the point of inducing bad health: "So hot he loved that at nighttime / He slept no more than does a nightingale" (Chaucer, 1963, lines 97–98).

Shakespeare is expert at such depictions, both tragic, as in *Romeo and Juliet*, and comic, as in *The Merchant of Venice*, in which Portia disguises herself as a young man and explains that she must

> . . . speak of frays
> Like a fine bragging youth, and tell quaint lies,
> How honorable ladies sought my love,
> Which I denying, they fell sick and died—
> (act 3, scene 4, lines 70–73)

Youths lose more than sleep and health to unbridled emotion. Reason is another victim, and sensibility, discretion, good taste, even character. Animal metaphors abound; thus, Shakespeare was moved to record that "for young hot colts being raged, do rage the more" (*Richard II*, act 2, scene 1, line 70). These images penetrate deeply into the literary and philosophical canons of Western thought, and throughout we find expressions of concern about youth's inclinations for getting into trouble, and advice on how to steer them away from it.

Clothed in the language and methods of modern science, this *risk-taking-as-trouble* orientation has organized a massive effort aimed at identifying the epidemiological, sociological, and developmental correlates of adolescents' risk behaviors. Over the longer haul, and in the tradition of the empiricist approach that frames this research, the goal is to pinpoint specific causes so that risk involvement can be predicted and controlled. It is well intended: Our children are coming of age in an era gripped by unparalleled teen pregnancy, drug addiction, suicide, and homicide. Beyond these more obvious consequences, their risks are attended by school dropout, welfare dependency, and incarceration. The desire to locate antecedent conditions is coupled tightly with a felt need to contain pressing social problems that are destroying the families, neighborhoods, and lives of youth.

Although this orientation has surely held the larger measure of our attentions, one can also identify a different point of view. This one, grounded more securely in developmental theory, and closer to the *risk-taking-as-opportunity* view, has it that adolescent problem behaviors are demonstrative of normative developmental concerns and processes. Thus conceived, risk-taking is as bound to issues of experimentation, autonomy, and identity development as it is to rebellion, trouble-making, and mischief.

Fornäs (1995) discusses a comparable distinction in a recent anthology of work focused on theoretical advances in the field of "youth culture studies" as conducted primarily at Stockholm University. In his introduction to the volume, he presents a distinction between two extremist sentiments toward youth that are ensconced, more or less implicitly, in contemporary research. One sees youths as trouble-makers and youth culture as degenerate and subversive. This, he argues, underlies traditional, problem-oriented research as it is carried out by "economically, politically, psychologically, or pedagogically oriented researchers" (p. 3). The other sentiment, just as extreme, softens all rough edges with the airbrush of romantic idealism. The best example here is the area of cultural studies, which is motivated by "optimistic curiosity about young people's creativity or by a sense of solidarity in the face of shared difficulties" (p. 3), and which, in true interdisciplinary fashion, has strong ties to hermeneutics, psychoanalysis, critical theory, structuralism, and semiotics.

RISK-TAKING AS OPPORTUNITY:
HEROES, ADVENTURES, AND THE
ACQUISITION OF SELF

As with the risk-taking-as-trouble orientation, the risk-taking-as-opportunity perspective also has roots in antiquity. In classical times, risks and adventures were construed as ordeals, tests of valor, virtue, strength, fidelity, and so forth, that were to be met and endured. Although this view dominated early European literature, a new vision of the hero emerged during the second half of the 18th century. The modern hero is one who takes on shape and character in consequence of risks and adventures; the modern hero *develops*. Remarkable events are not encountered by simple happenstance, but actively sought for their capacity to challenge and educate. It seems, then, that risks were not *taken*, exactly, until fairly recently. Part of the following chapter is devoted to the historical emergence of the hero and how it was shaped by changing conceptions of identity, development, and experience. For now I mean only to draw out the two cultural–historical casts responsible for our conflicted and ambivalent understanding of the adventures and misadventures of youth. John Dewey brings them into sharper relief when he describes our usual metric for the "goodness" of children as "the amount of trouble they make for grownups, which means of course the amount they deviate from adult habits and expectations. Yet by way of expiation we envy children their love of new experiences, their intentness in extracting the last drop of significance from each situation, their vital seriousness in things that to us are outworn" (1922, p. 99).

By Dewey's reading, the happier moments of children's exploration and study are just as lively and significant as those that are querulous and potentially hurtful. Jane Addams (1910) argued that the latter often overshadow the former, and obscure their common connections. At the turn of the century, she devoted a book to her experiences working with adolescents who arrived in America's industrial centers in unprecedented numbers. She wrote of their "quest for adventure" as a natural developmental period, and the source of their unflagging energy, enthusiasm, and zealous pursuit of novelty. But for many, newly arrived in a city illprepared to receive them, it was also their undoing: "The young people are overborne by their own undirected and misguided energies. A mere temperamental outbreak in a brief period of obstreperousness exposes a promising boy to arrest and imprisonment, an accidental combination of circumstances too complicated and overwhelming to be coped with by an immature mind, condemns a growing lad to a criminal career" (1910, pp. 51–52).

Undirected, fevered, tempted, reckless: These are the essences of youth, the natural consequences of emotion unfurled and unchecked by higher mental functions. Surviving centuries of scrutiny by poets and philosophers, these essences remain unparched even by the hot lights of modern science. Indeed, psychological theories of adolescent development have from the beginning drawn breath from them. G. Stanley Hall (1904), author of the first comprehensive compendium of adolescent psychology (its title was nothing less than *Adolescence: Its Psychology and Its Relations to Physiology, Anthropology, Sociology, Sex, Crime, Religion, and Education*) adopted a biogenetic and recapitulationist posture. Believing that the development of each individual is a fast-forward replay of the evolution of the entire species—that ontogeny recapitulates phylogeny—Hall saw the restlessness, recklessness, and eagerness of adolescence as marking a turning point. In his view, it is only with the advent of adolescence that the individual for the first time breaks through the predetermined phyletic structure to act in ways that are truly individual, unique, and agentic: truly human, by Hall's lights. Adolescence heralds the end of the lockstep, phylogenetic sequence, and is accordingly a period of unprecedented flexibility and plasticity of thought, feeling, and behavior. Our best response, as parents, educators, or persons in other roles that minister to the well-being of children, is to give adolescents a loose rein and thereby enable their personal exploration and experimentation. Seeing in all of this an agenda for policy and education, Hall reasoned that because adolescents are by their very nature primed to be inspired, we ought to take steps to inspire them. History, he argued, ought to be the study of heroes, science the study of cosmic forces. Hall was the first to insist on a "moratorium" for youth, a time out from responsibility and obligation in order that they might explore in the freest possible manner the world and discover their places within it.

In modern scientific circles, the risk-taking-as-opportunity perspective can perhaps trace its lineage to Hall's grandiose beginnings. There is at least strong evidence of historical continuity: Hall's theory of moratoruim; Addams's report of youth's fitful "quest for adventure"; Erik Erikson's thesis of the adolescent "craving for locomotion."

> The most widespread expression of the discontented search of youth is the craving for locomotion, whether expressed in a general "being on the go," "tearing after something," or "running around"; or in locomotion proper, as in vigorous work, in absorbing sports, in rapt dancing, in shiftless *Wanderschaft*, and in the employment and misuse of speedy animals and machines. But it also finds expression through participation in the movements of the day (whether the riots of a local commotion or the parades and campaigns of major ideological forces), if they only appeal to the need for feeling "moved" and for feeling essential in moving something along toward an open future. (Erikson, 1963, p. 11)

Erikson's main thesis was that "locomotion" constitutes a form of excessive experimentation, of testing the limits of one's self, of exploring its multiple possibilities, especially its relations to society. All of this speaks to a search for "some durability in change," and for those who find it, a sense of identity interdependent with community and history. Thus, the concept of the "psychosocial moratorium" (popularized by Erikson, 1968), which continues to exert considerable force in modern identity development theory, is nothing less than a codification of the idea that adolescents engage in a period of experimentation from which they emerge with a foothold on who they will become. But whereas the risk-taking-as-trouble orientation has harnessed the energy of a generation of researchers bent on preventing adolescent risk-taking, the perspective put forth by Hall, Addams, and Erikson, and those of their ilk has been less seminal. Only recently have investigators considered the possibility that risk involvement may have positive consequences for psychosocial development. Baumrind, for example, referred to some risk-taking behaviors as "the pursuit of opportunities for self-transcendent challenge" (1987, p. 98). Those sympathetic to this emerging point of view are making claims that pot smoking, wild driving, early sexual intimacy, and so forth, have strategic roles in achieving social status, demonstrating autonomy, and hedging boredom and anxiety. Jessor (1992) argued that the reason adolescent risk involvement is so intractable to change is because it serves these ordinary developmental goals so well. In fact, in failing to provide resources that would promote alternative behaviors, the "Just Say No!" campaign dismisses the functional utility of adolescents' risks (more on this below), and guarantees that it will provide nothing more than ineffectual rhetoric with which to decorate car bumpers.[1]

CONCEPTUALIZING CAUSES OF ADOLESCENT RISK-TAKING

Despite the inference that adolescents take risks because they are adolescents (which we have no control over, naturally), the search continues for more local causes that would account for individual differences and provide some guidelines for prevention and control by allowing us to predict one's risk for risks. But as McCord (1990) amply demonstrates in her comprehensive review of the social/community factors, biogenetic susceptibilities, personality traits, and parent and peer influences, we have found nothing that can be described legitimately as a causal link. It seems, moreover, that a distressing number of treatment programs appear to do more harm than good, and to date, the most promising preventive measure appears to be a program for *preschoolers* (see also Zigler, Taussig, & Black, 1992).[2]

It could be argued that part of the problem lies in a sluggishness to adopt methodologies acknowledging that risk behaviors are multiply determined. We can envision this argument as insisting on the possibility that different causes (e.g., family or peer influences)

---

[1]To be honest, the risk-as-opportunity claims made here have little genuine empirical support, probably owing to the recency with which researchers have taken seriously this alternative point of view. A noteworthy exception is a study by Shedler and Block (1990), which found that adolescents who experimented with drugs were better adjusted than those who used drugs frequently or not at all. It is important to point out, as Shedler and Block do, that the study does not show experimentation to cause or promote good mental health, but to be one of its signs, tokens, or symptoms.

[2]This particular preschool project encourages family involvement, and its long-term success is consistent with a body of literature that indicates strong associations between family identification and parenting practices, and adolescent delinquency (Baumrind, 1989; Kandel & Lesser, 1972; Shedler & Block, 1990).

might underlie similar risks, or that a single risk might be caused by a confluence of interacting factors. This argument has a good deal of intuitive appeal. It seems entirely sensible that one teenager might smoke his first joint to demonstrate his daring, whereas another might be looking to escape anxiety brought on by an unhappy family situation. Or consider the young women in Los Angeles who have sex with HIV-infected young men as part of their initiation into gangs. Here, the risk is multiply determined—the young women demonstrate their commitment to the group, but also gain the protection of the gang in an increasingly dangerous city.

Related to the argument that the correspondence between risks and their causes is something other than one-to-one are the appeals to acknowledge the correspondence between risks. It is now well established that adolescents who are taking risks are taking them, in all likelihood, in a variety of domains. Smoking, drinking, drug use, sexual precocity, and dangerous driving are all of a piece. Yet risk involvement is rarely studied this way; research moves instead through one domain at a time. Jessor (1992), among others (e.g., Bell & Bell, 1993; Irwin, 1990; Kegeles, Millstein, & Adler, 1987), is concerned that this "problem of the week approach" obscures the extent to which risks cause other risks, the logic of which is inherent in public service announcements that warn, "Get high, get stupid, get AIDS."

Finally, the recent move to establish a general consensus on the definition of "problem behavior," "reckless behavior," or "risk-taking" can be seen as another sort of effort to sweep away the ambiguities that hang between the behaviors themselves and the factors that cause them. Most now agree that these sorts of activities are volitional, purposive, goal oriented, and carry potential for harm. Lopes (1987) reminds us that, technically speaking, "risk" refers to decision-making situations in which various probabilities are attached to the possible outcomes of future events. Results from several studies indicate, in fact, that adolescents are very much aware that their risk behaviors are indeed risky (e.g., DiBlasio, 1986; Irwin & Millstein, 1987; Klintzer, Rossiter, Gruenewald, & Balinsky, 1987), prompting many investigators to call for a reappraisal. In particular, there is growing support for the possibility that adolescent risk-taking is a reasonably rational and thoughtful process that differs hardly at all from the decision-making processes of adults (e.g., Furby & Beyth-Marom, 1992; Gardner, 1993; Lopes, 1993).

Although defining risk-taking as purposeful activity has helped to focus attention on the decision making processes through which teenagers identify and attach evaluative weight to the potential consequences of their behaviors, others are calling for a more finely honed taxonomy. Researchers have discussed the importance of separating getting drunk or smoking the occasional joint from crack addiction, for example. After all, experimenting with alcohol and marijuana (inhaling or not) is typical of American youth, whereas crack addiction occurs less often and carries more serious consequences. We are dealing in the first case with behaviors that are considered normative, exploratory, or transitional to adult status and functioning, whereas the second case is an example of behaviors that are clearly health compromising, destructive, and pathogenic. Speaking for many, Irwin (1993) argues that "a major problem for investigators and clinicians is to distinguish between normal transitional risk-taking behaviors that are developmentally enhancing and those same behaviors that, by their frequency or intensity, are pathological expressions for which there is little evidence of secondary gain for the teenager" (p. 12).

The distinction between these classes of risk gives some coherence to the enormous literature concerned with adolescents' risk-taking and problem behaviors. It also gives contemporary form to the history of our ambivalence. We now have a classification system (albeit a simple one) that allows us to address adolescents' risks as both constructive and undesirable, as developmentally enhancing and impeding, as opportunity and trouble. However, still framed within the empirical–analytic tradition, the assumption is that we are dealing with apples and oranges, that different causal mechanisms are operating, and could be identified, if the two cases were not conflated empirically. Already movement is discernible among clinicians and personality theorists who would annex the truly problematic, deep-seated, and pathological, and set it apart from the more mundane, bread-and-butter variety of risks observed in most normally developing adolescents. However, there are reasons to believe that simply increasing the number of variables studied, or narrowing the focus of investigation to some agreed-upon set of behaviors would gain little purchase in specifying causal linkages. In light of extreme ethnic and community variations in what constitutes problem behavior, definition by consensus seems unlikely, if not inappropriate. For example, crossing the street can be risky business if you're trespassing onto the forbidden turf of a neighborhood gang, and becoming a pregnant teen in a neighborhood in which it is normative to do so puts a wrinkle in any pat declaration that such behavior is delinquent or deviant. This is not to dramatize the risk of daily living, or to diminish the personal, social, and economic costs of teen pregnancy. It is meant, instead, to call attention to the poor track record of efforts to understand adolescents' risks within a cause–effect paradigm, and to invite an exploration of different methodological paths.

Interpretive methodology departs intentionally from the cause–effect language of the empiricist tradition for the purpose of presenting a more "interpretive" (Dilthey 1900/1976; Taylor, 1985) or "reconstructive" (Habermas, 1979) approach. In contrast to prevailing perspectives that focus on youth's *disposition* for risk involvement as a natural consequence of separable and preexisting causes (e.g., cognitive immaturities, bad neighborhoods, undue peer influence, lackadaisical or overbearing parenting), I am here concerned with youth's *composition* of risks as artifice and aesthetics. I view them, in other words, as interpretive activity, as meaningful action, as experience. This perspective carries with it an entirely distinct set of assumptions regarding the causal connections between risks and the contexts in which they are realized. Within the empiricist tradition, the connections are understood to be mechanical and directional; risks are outcome variables, *effects* of independent, antecedent *causes*. Within the interpretive paradigm, however, they are internal and systemic, held together by connections that are formal, logical, or conceptual, rather than statistical or empirical (Lightfoot & Valsiner, 1992; Valsiner, 1987).

The potential value of focusing on the meanings of risk experience for those who have them and those who participate within the same interpretive community is underscored by a recent comment made by Jeffrey Arnett (1992). In criticizing Jessor's (1992) argument that adolescents' problem behaviors function as transition markers toward more mature status, he remarked that "no evidence has been presented by Jessor or others to support it," and that "[p]erhaps it would be useful to interview adolescents about their reasons for engaging in reckless/problem/risk behavior. Do they state or imply the desire for a more mature status as one of their motivations?" (p. 404). As we shall see, the answer to his question is in fact an unequivocal "yes," but what is particularly striking in his challenge, and what makes it entirely justified, is that after centuries of worry and concern and years of empirical scrutiny, we know very little about the meanings implicit in adolescent risk behaviors.

STEPS TOWARD A DIFFERENT AGENDA

Discussing adolescent risk involvement in interpretive terms is not entirely without precedent, at least, there is a history of thought and research that points in this general direction. What follows is a highly selective review of theory and research that can be seen to converge on a general perspective that views risk-taking as a form of activity relevant to cultural development. The first family of approaches permits an analysis of the social processes and functions of risk-taking; the second encourages a form of interpretation that is more structural and systemic.

Social Process and Functional Approaches

Part of this approach comes from efforts to link risk behavior to social norms and peer expectations. Studies of alcohol safety courses, for example, have shown that although such courses increase students' *knowledge* about alcohol risk and safety, they have little impact on students' *attitudes* or driving while intoxicated (DWI) *behaviors* (e.g., McKnight, Preusser, Psotka, Katz, & Edwards, 1979). A similar perplexity obtains with regard to adolescent girls' contraceptive knowledge and behavior: being informed of the facts of things—how to get pregnant and how to avoid it—is a poor predictor of whether or not young women will use contraceptives (Cvetkovich, Grote, Bjorseth, & Sarkissian, 1975; Gerrard, McCann, & Fortini, 1983, cited in Arnett, 1992). Likewise, Kegeles, Adler, and Irwin (1988, cited in Furby & Beyth-Marom, 1992) found no relation between adolescents' intention to use condoms, and their knowledge of condoms as effective in preventing pregnancy and venereal diseases.

Rather, the intention to use condoms was associated with beliefs about condoms as easy to use, acceptable to peers, and interfering with spontaneity.

Findings of ethnic and gender differences also implicate social norms and expectations as potential mediators of risk behavior. Klintzer et al. (1987), for example, found that perceived deviance of DWI was a strong predictor of self-reported DWI, and that perceived deviance varied considerably across Hispanic, black, and white ethnic groups. In the same vein, Millstein and Irwin (1987) suggested gender differences in the *content* of reported risks: males were more likely to have driven under the influence of alcohol or other drugs, whereas females were more likely to have ridden in a car with an impaired driver.

Although several of the investigators cited above have invoked social learning processes, DiBlasio (1986) has been the most articulate spokesperson for social learning constructs, including differential association, imitation, and reinforcement. He argues that through differential association, adolescents are exposed to and identify with various groups that influence the development of normative definitions of each member, including personal attitudes and beliefs about rules, laws, and values, which guide the individual in making choices to act in law-abiding or -violating ways. His survey of more than 1,000 16- and 17-year-olds indicated that differential peer association (i.e., frequency, duration, intensity of relationship with peers who drink while intoxicated, or who ride with an impaired driver) was the strongest predictor of DWI. Klintzer and his colleagues (1987) also found a strong relationship between DWI and peer drinking practices; and Jessor, Chase, and Donovan (1980) found that friends' approval and the availability of potent models were the strongest predictors of a number of adolescent problem behaviors.

Sociologists have taken a leading role in emphasizing the importance of social processes in mediating adolescent risk-taking and problem behavior. Much of their work focuses on the role of deviant peer group norms in regulating the behavior of group members. Sociological studies of delinquent groups, for example, indicate that norms of deviance and aggression are shared between group members, and provide a basis for interaction, affiliation, and friendship (e.g., Giordano, Cernkovich, & Pugh, 1986). A history of research on adolescent drug and alcohol use echo these findings (Dembo, Schmeidler, & Burgos, 1979; Kandel, 1978; Hubba, Wingard, & Bentler, 1979): Individual and collective norms regarding drug use may determine the *selection* of particular individuals as friends, and also the *maintenance and stability* of drug and alcohol use within groups (e.g., Britt & Campbell, 1977; Kandel, 1978). For example, a longitudinal study of marijuana use among friendship pairs showed that preexisting drug use was a source of interpersonal attraction that influenced the formation of friendships, and that similarities in drug use increased over time within stable relationships (Kandel, 1978). Kandel's work suggests that processes of selection and socialization operate jointly to augment behavioral, psychological, and ideological similarities among group members.

In addition to exploring the mechanisms that render problem behaviors functional *within* particular groups or relationships, some care has been taken to acknowledge that peer groups function within larger communities. The work of Cairns and his colleagues (Cairns, Cairns, Neckerman, Gest, & Gariépy, 1988) is an example. In their studies of peer groups and deviant behavior they found that highly aggressive adolescents cluster together into social groups that are organized comparably to nonaggressive groups (see also Hubba et al., 1979). However, individuals in aggressive groups were found to be unpopular in the social network at large. It was speculated that individuals within aggressive cliques may be more likely to drop out of school due to rejection or expulsion, and have difficulty becoming integrated into the larger community. Additonal evidence for the relative social isolation of groups engaged in marginal risk behaviors comes from a study of high school and college students' perceptions of common crowd types (e.g., brains, jocks, druggies, populars, toughs; Brown, Lohr, & Trujillo, 1990). Students reported that druggies and toughs were more likely to be socially disruptive and to hang out in out of the way places, and were less likely to be involved in extracurricular activities, compared to individuals in less deviant crowds.

Another well-articulated functional approach is found is some of the collected works edited by Silbereisen, Eyferth, and Rudinger (1986). Their volume entitled *Development as Action in Context* is arguably the first comprehesive commentary on the "normalcy" of adolescent problem behavior. The collection of papers reflects a general commitment to developmental theory that places self-regu-lated action at centerstage. Silbereisen et al. summarize it as follows: "Development is seen as the outcome of a person's own intentional, goal-oriented action aimed at adjusting individual goals and poten-tials to contextual demands and opportunties. Such action produces not only change in the individual, but change in the context of de-velopment as well. The contextual changes thus induced continually provide opportunities for new action aimed at further development" (p. 4).

From this perspective, problem behaviors (smoking pot, for ex-ample) and positive behaviors (having an independent opinion) may be "functional equivalents," depending on the underlying goal structure (e.g., demonstrating one's independence). Likewise, similar behaviors may serve different goals and, therefore, have different functions. In either case, the point to be made is that risk-taking may be illuminated by acknowledging the agentic qualities of the adoles-cent whose risk-taking is both future oriented and goal directed.

Jessor's early prospective longitudinal work is an excellent ex-ample of how adolescent risk-taking may be advantageously placed within a developmental–functional conceptual framework (e.g., Jes-sor & Jessor, 1975). In essence, adolescent problem behavior was un-derstood as a "syndrome" that represents part of the adolescent lifestyle. From this perspective problem behavior constitutes a means of accomplishing age-typical goals—peer group entry and adult status achievment, for example. Supporting their position is evidence that the onset of drinking appears as part of a more gener-al behavioral pattern that includes placing greater value on inde-pendence relative to achievement, peer (as opposed to parent) orien-tation, and increased social criticism. Furthermore, this pattern was found to constitute a transition away from a level of development in which behavior is characteristically conforming and conventional. Jessor and Jessor argued that alcohol consumption represents the adolescent's attempt to cross the status boundary from childhood to adulthood. Construed as a "transition-marker," its appearence at early ages may actually reflect precocious social development (see also Stacey & Davies, 1970).

The social-psychological perspective developed by Jessor and Jessor led to a recommendation for social-psychological interventions. In particular, they argued that teen-drinking prevention may be facilitated by efforts to dissolve the culturally derived meaning attached to alcohol use as a symbol of adult status. This, in conjunction with Silbereisen's insights, bears directly on the utility of framing "problem behaviors" within a context of meaning. For example, Silbereisen and his colleagues have argued that adolescent substance use may serve a variety of functions, depending on intra- and extrapersonal circumstances. They compiled a lengthy, but probably still incomplete, list of such circumstances:

> Taking substances (a) can represent an instance of excessive and ritualized behaviors, (b) it may indicate a lack of self-control, (c) could serve as a means to deviate purposively from norms, (d) is a specific developmental task, considering that controlled, ceremonial use is positively sanctioned, (e) may express an age-typical life-style, and (f) can indicate atempts to cope with helplessness and stress. (reported in English in Silbereisen & Eyferth, 1986, p. 8)

Along similar lines, Lastovicka, Murry, Joachimsthaler, Bhalla, and Scheurich (1987), identified five different types of risk-takers: delinquents, party-goers, sensation seekers, machoists, and dissatisfied. Although recognizing the contributions of decision-making processes and rational cost–benefit analysis, they made the point that risk behaviors are significantly motivated by their symbolic value in maintaining one's concept of self as, for example, a macho person or a sensation seeker. The innovation here is the emphasis on self-concept, and the relationship between individuals and their social groups, that is, the relational contexts in which one's actions have meaning. Risky behaviors are not effective symbols unless they are recognized as such by others. Thus, understanding adolescent risk-taking lies at least in part in understanding the collective and personal meanings of risk behaviors. This takes us beyond strictly functional and social process accounts, which emphasize the weight that accrues to risk behavior by virtue of its effectiveness in acheiving certain personal or interpersonal rewards or reinforcements, or its value as a means to goal attainment. We are called upon to reckon with the way in which risk behavior defines one's sense of self, and one's relationships with others.

Structural and Systems Approaches:
Self-Development in Relational Contexts

There is a long history of interest in the role of relationships in the development of self, especially the development of self that takes place during adolescence. Developmentalists interested in adolescent peer relational processes, some of whom were mentioned above, have taken leads from classic studies in social psychology and sociology. The Robbers Cave experiment of Sherif and his colleagues (Sherif, Harvey, White, Hood, & Sherif, 1961), for example, has had a tremendous impact on conceptualizations of the formation of peer group norms. And Moreno's (1934) and Dunphy's (1963) inroads into the sociometry and structure of groups laid a foundation for devising methodological tools with which to describe group characteristics and organization (see Hartup, 1983, for a historical overview).

The conceptual position of Sherif and his colleagues (Sherif et al., 1961; Sherif & Sherif, 1964) was that social groups constitute frames of reference for individuals who act within them. Group norms, or standards of conduct, that delimit the actions of members, serve as anchor points in structuring the "perceptual field." From this perspective, the group is less an objective collection of individuals than a psychological organization of each member's experiences: Joint activity and participation in social groups leads to the generation and instantiation of group norms that structure and give meaning to experiences.

In a theoretical paper entitled "Reference Groups as Perspectives," Shibutani (1955) elaborated Sherif's ideas and proposed that reference groups arise through the internalization of norms. In his words, "they constitute the structure of expectations imputed to some audience for whom one organizes his conduct" (p. 565). He argued that reference groups are a product of social interactions and communication. People approach one another from particular perspectives, which are confirmed, reinforced, denied, and thereby transformed in the course of interpersonal transactions. It is through social participation, then, that perspectives become shared and internalized. All social groupings, regardless of size, composition, structure, or overlap may become reference groups through members' participation in common communication channels. Reference group theory, according to Shibutani, is particularly crucial for understanding individuals in modern mass societies—those marked by a diversity and multiplicity of communication channels and opportunities for participation:

> In the analysis of the behavior of men in mass societies the crucial problem is that of ascertaining how a person defines the situation, which perspective he uses in arriving at such a definition, and who constitutes the audience whose responses provide the necessary confirmation and support for his position. This calls for focusing attention upon the expectations the actor imputes to others, the communication channels in which he participates, and his relations with those with whom he identifies himself. (p. 569)

The major focus of reference group theory, then, is on the subjective aspects of group life: how the individual organizes social interaction and experience such that norms are internalized and the group becomes a frame of reference for organizing future action.

While reference group theory has been particularly influential in sociological circles, modern theories of self and social relations owe much of their inspiration and direction to the early work of George Herbert Mead, who argued that self-development is all about changes in role-taking abilties. Role-taking is a deliberate act to "call out" in oneself responses that would be called out in the "other." The self–other connectedness established through role-taking is integral to social functioning. Mead claimed, in fact, that people distinguish themselves as members of society to the extent that they permit the attitudes of others to take control of their own immediate expressions (Mead, 1934, p. 223). But the highest form of social functioning (and the highest level of self development) is observed when actions are guided by the "generalized other"—the organized system of all group members' perspectives in relation to the self. As Mead (1934) articulated, construction of the generalized other is a developmental and personal process:

> [T]he organized structure of every individual self within the human social process of experience and behavior reflects and is constituted by the organized relational pattern of that process as a whole; but

each individual self-structure reflects and is constituted by a different aspect or perspective of this relational pattern, because each reflects this relational pattern from its own unique standpoint, so that the common social origin and constitution of individual selves and their structures does not preclude wide individual differences and variation among them or contradict the peculiar and more or less distinctive individuality which each of them in fact possesses. . . . The individual, as we have seen, is continually reacting back against this society. Every adjustment involves some sort of change in the community to which the individual adjusts himself. (pp. 234–235)

As is eminently apparent here, Mead acknowledged the active nature both of individuals and of the communities in which they act. Moreover, the general process of the individual's "adjustments against society," and the organization of adjustments into structures that reflect and are constituted by social patterns, is implicated in the ability to participate in a community of practices, as well as the ability eventually to take one's self as an object of thought. Although some well-argued criticism has been leveled against Mead's emphasis on the developmental relevance of dyadic interaction as opposed to semiotic activity (e.g., Lee & Hickmann, 1983), the twofold process, or dual genesis, of participation/identification and reflection/critique is at the core of contemporary interpretive approaches, as will be discussed later.

The connection between social action and self-reflection was not missed by Inhelder and Piaget's account of the development of thinking and self (1958). They close their book *The Growth of Logical Thinking from Childhood to Adolescence* with a chapter devoted to the relationship between formal thought and the enactment of adult roles. In step with their overall research agenda, they discussed the conceptual links between adolescent hypothetical reasoning, self-reflection, and a commitment to future possibilities. The ability to think in terms of possibilities, in addition to actualities, and the ability to reflect on the self in relation to future possibilities, permit the construction of "life programs":

[T]he adolescent is no longer content to live the interindiviudal relations offered by his immediate surroundings or to use his intelligence to solve the problems of the moment. Rather, he is motivated also to take his place in the adult social framework, and with this aim he tends to participate in the ideas, ideals, and ideologies of a wider group through the medium of a number of verbal symbols to which he was indifferent as a child. (p. 341)

In the course of adopting adult roles, the adolescent reflects on and organizes his or her future activity in relation to adult society. But from the structural develomental position of Inhelder and Piaget (1958), prior to the emergence of formal thought during adolescence, self–society relations are not fully differentiated and integrated, and the child is unable to organize a personal life program that coheres pragmatically with adult society.

The contention that adolescents become increasingly able to envision interdependent relations between themselves and the social system in which they will participate has been supported by Trommsdorff's studies of adolescents' future time orientation (1986). Future orientation was described as a cognitive–motivational complex: "the anticipation and evaluation of the future self in interaction with the environment" (p. 122). Building her conceptual base, she cited work that found that adolescents structure their futures more complexly, and in step with general (formal operational) cognitive developments: Time perspectives extend more into the future, become increasingly realistic, and the causes of future events are taken into account. What this perspective has to offer to our understanding of risk-taking is suggested in Trommsdorff's comparative study of delinquent drug users and nonusers. The future orientation of users was found to be more pessimistic with respect to social acceptance and integration; it was less extended in time, with higher expectations of fearful outcomes. Trommsdorff held up these data as an indication of a vicious circle between future orientation (toward further drug use and continuing social failure) and environmental conditions that reinforce exactly those negative anticipations through continuing social sanctions and disapproval.

The structural immaturity attending the onset of formal operations—the lack of self–society integration—is also observed in adolescents' inclinations to form life programs consistent with reformed (ideal) worlds rather than actual (probabilistic) worlds:

The indefinite extension of powers of thought made possible by the new instruments of propositional logic at first is conducive to failure to distinguish between the ego's new and unpredicted capacities and the social or cosmic universe to which they are applied. In other words, the adolescent goes through a phase in which he attributes an unlimited power to his own thoughts so that the dream of a glorious future or of transforming the world through Ideas seems to be not only fantasy but also an effective action which in itself modifies the empirical world. This is obviously a form of cognitive egocentrism. (Inhelder & Piaget, 1958, pp. 345–346)

Adolescent egocentrism, according to Inhelder and Piaget (1958), is expressed in the "idealistic crisis" or "crisis of juvenile originality," in which adolescents enthusiastically embrace and then abandon successive sets of ideals, moral causes, or visions of a more perfect world. Such cycles of enchantment and disenchantment are thus symptomatic of cognitive limitations: The adolescent fails to recognize the interdependent and integrated nature of self in relation to society. Consequently, the self is believed invested with unlimited possibilities. The reader will recognize in this description of "cognitive egocentrism" the historical stepping stone to David Elkind's (1978) popular construct of "adolescent egocentrism," and its subcategories of the imaginary audience, apparent hypocrisy, pseudostupidity, and the personal fable. The last of these, the personal fable, has been suspected of underlying a lot of adolescent problem behaviors (e.g., Arnett, 1992). Elkind writes:

> The personal fable then accounts, in part at least, for a variety of perplexing and troubling behaviors exhibited by the young teenager. It helps account for what appears to be self-destructive behavior but in fact results from a belief that the young person is special and shielded from harm. "It can happen to others, not to me." And the personal fable also accounts for the young adolescent's self-deprecating and self-aggrandizing behavior. In general, personal fable behavior begins to diminish as young people begin to develop friendships in which intimacies are shared. Once young people begin to share their personal feelings and thoughts, they discover that they are less unique and special than they thought. In addition, the sense of loneliness in being special and apart from everyone else diminishes as the personal fable becomes less obtrusive. (p. 132)

In contrast to how Piagetian theory is often portrayed as "reducing" all developments to internal structural–cognitive changes (but, cf. Youniss & Smollar, 1985), social relations, as Elkind reiterates above, are held accountable for the adolescent's eventual decentration (Inhelder & Piaget, 1958; Piaget, 1965/1995). It is in the context of the peer group and the occupational world that adolescents test their personal ideologies against those of others, and discover their fragilities: "[S]ocial contact is what brings about consciousness of the self" (Piaget, 1965/1995, p. 223).

That peer groups and peer relations provide a likely context for adolescent decentration is also at the heart of Selman's (1980) work on social perspective-taking, which has been elaborated recently to account for adolescent risk behavior (Levitt & Selman, 1996). In the model presented, risk-taking behavior is illuminated according to a dimension of "personal meaning"—a developing capacity to appreciate how one's pattern of risk behavior is embedded in one's own life history and social relationships. The authors call attention to how the development of self-reflection, perspective coordination, and affective engagement contribute to the meanings attached to risk behaviors. They argue, moreover, that increasing maturity in these domains acts ultimately as a preventive factor.

Both the functional and the structural approaches to adolescent risk-taking can be oriented within an interpretive perspective. As discussed above, interpretive and empiricist methodologies present separate agendas for studying human development, and proceed from incompatible epistemological assumptions (Lightfoot & Folds-Bennett, 1991). The latter has generally dominated developmental psychology, but for the reasons described above, has provided only disappointing explanations of adolescent risk-taking. However, interpretive methodologies will be shown to hold promise for deciphering the *meanings* of these experiences for those who have them and those who participate within the same intepretive community. As discussed by Gaskins, Miller, and Corsaro (1992), interpretive methods of data collection and analysis are intended to search out "concrete" universals as opposed to "statistical generalizations," and are more focused on establishing "cultural validity" than reliability. By the same logic, Geertz (1983) argues that interpretive explanation looks less for the sort of thing "that connects planets and pendulums and more for the sort that connects chrysanthemums and swords":

> Interpretive explanation—and it is a form of explanation, not just
> exalted glossography—trains its attention on what institutions, ac-
> tions, images, utterances, events, customs, all the usual objects of so-
> cial–scientific interest, mean to those whose institutions, actions, cus-
> toms, and so on they are. As a result, it issues not laws like Boyle's,
> or forces like Volta's, or mechanisms like Darwin's but constructions
> like Buckhardt's, Weber's, or Freud's systematic unpacking of the
> conceptual world in which *condotiere*, Calvinists, or paranoids live.
> (pp. 19–20)

I mean to argue that taking risks occupies a position of privilege in the repertoire of human experience and development.
Defining risk involvement as interpretive activity takes us some distance, I think, in understanding why adolescents pursue it with such
devotion. In a manner strikingly similar to many psychologists' ex-
coriations of the "Just Say No!" campaign, a teenager expressed the
following view of "peer pressure" and the efforts of adults to protect
him from it:

> "There's all this crap about being accepted into a group and
> struggling and making an effort to make friends and not be-
> ing comfortable about your own self-worth as a human being.
> . . . [But] the idea of peer pressure is a lot of bunk. What I
> heard about peer pressure all the way through school is that
> someone is going to walk up to me and say 'Here, drink this
> and you'll be cool.' It wasn't like that at all. You go some-
> where and everyone else would be doing it and you'd think,
> 'Hey, everyone else is doing it and they seem to be having a
> good time—now why wouldn't I do this?' In that sense, the
> preparation of the powers that be, the lessons that they tried
> to drill into me, they were completely off. They have no idea
> what we're up against."

In the pages that follow, I hope, at the very least, to convey
some sense of what they are up against. In the course of analyzing
the interviews, I will address the teenagers' definitions of risk, their
motives for risk involvement, and their understanding the relevance
of risk-taking for adolescents. I will discuss the stories they told, both

general and specific, about risks and adventures shared with friends, as well as their interpretations of risks taken by hypothetical characters. First, however, I will attempt to illuminate a logic, both historical and theoretical, in which adolescents' risks are seen as devices for constituting self and cultural identity.

CHAPTER 3

The Interpretive Turn

Where is the center of events, the common standpoint
around which they revolve and which gives them cohesion? In
order that something like cohesion, something like causality,
that some kind of meaning might ensue and that it can in
some way be narrated, the historian must invent units, a hero,
a nation, an idea, and he must allow to happen to this
invented unity what has in reality happened to the nameless.
                                            —HERMANN HESSE

By the lights of modern interpretive theory, we are all Hesse's historian. We discover our selves and our world, and make them coherent and communicable through interpretive activity. Thoughts, experiences, intentions, memories, desires, and all of our other
intelligibles are inventions of our own design and construction.

The thesis that our interpretations express and constitute who
we are and what we know has been broadcast within philosophy,
psychology, anthropology, sociology, political science—within virtually every discipline that concerns itself with the organization of human activity and social praxis. This multidisciplinary "interpretive
turn" has been taken from the well-traveled road of *hermeneutics*, a
paradigm associated historically with the exegesis of literary, especially religious, documents. In allegiance to this tradition, human interaction and culture are construed as readable *text* (e.g., Dilthey,
1900/1976; Gadamer, 1975; Heidegger, 1927/1976; Ricoeur,
1972; Taylor, 1985). This basic notion has been articulated to include three basic assumptions: (1) that texts and their congeners—
narrative, autobiography, voice—impose coherence on reality
rather than correspond to it directly (they are inventive); (2) that
writing a text is an inherently social, dialogical, or semiotic affair;
and (3) that texts are constructed and reconstructed in and over

time, and carry their histories forward through time. This constitutes the triumvirate of modern interpretive theory. As I shall try to make clear, it also maps out the primary concerns of contemporary developmental psychology, at least as it has been pursued from within the organismic paradigm (Valsiner, 1994a). Each of the three assumptions made its debut in the writings of some of the major historical figures in the discipline, including Kurt Lewin, Heinz Werner, Lev Vygotsky, Piaget, and Freud, but they were unable to sustain much of the initial momentum. The intellectual climate of the time espoused not only different and incompatible assumptions, but assumptions that captured the imagination of a generation bearing witness to the birth of the machine age—assumptions that cohered with that new age and played more than a bit part in making it possible. In recent years, however, the three assumptions of the organismic perspective have been exhumed, revived, and invigorated by advances in interpretive theory.

THREE ASSUMPTIONS

Until the early years of the 20th century, the hermeneutic paradigm (and science in general) was dominated by a "naive realism" or "objectivism" in which texts were understood to have unique and determinable meanings existing independently of their interpretations; they contained truths, sometimes divine, waiting to be discovered by the careful or the faithful. This particular form of realism recedes into the shadows of interpretationism at the turn of the century as reflected in Heidegger's (1927/1976) argument that text and reader are conjoined within a circle-structure of understanding. Following the conceptual evolution leading from Heidegger to Gadamer and Wittgenstein (all principals in the interpretive turn of events), the emerging interpretationism is seen to settle around the notion that all understanding proceeds from the "positive prejudices," "prejudgments," or "fore-conceptions" of the interpreter's time and epoch. Connolly and Keutner (1988, p. 18) convey Heidegger's position that "we are not simply entities or 'objects in the world,' rather we find ourselves 'hurled' into a network of institutions, purposes, plans, tools, implements, et al., toward all of which our basic stance is 'understanding.' . . . [A]t this level things such as chairs or trees are not regarded as 'physical objects,' but rather as implements in, or constituents of, the plans, purposes, etc., of our lives."

Advancing Dilthey's metaphor of the circle, Heidegger means to embrace the fullness of lived experience left out of abstract cognitive models. His most visible target is Husserl's hierarchical model, which gives pride of place to the mind's capacity for bracketing experience so as to contemplate it over time (Hirsch, 1976; Lightfoot, in press-b). Although the clash of metaphors—the circle against the hierarchy—has important historic and heuristic value, classical constructivist theories in psychology come very close to presenting a more integrative perspective. Expressing similar sentiments about the individual's active part in the construction of reality, Piaget, for example, writes that "[j]ust as, when a rabbit eats cabbage, he is not changed into cabbage but, on the contrary, the cabbage is changed into rabbit, so in all action or praxis, the subject is not absorbed in the object, but the object is used and 'included' as relative to the subject's actions" (1972, p. 71).

Vygotsky's theory of psychological development is similar in its constructivist epistemology, and has become recently popular in North American circles because of its outwardly sociocultural concerns (Rieber & Carton, 1987; Valsiner, 1988). Vygotsky set himself the task of explicating the development of higher mental functions, and setting them apart, in structure and origin, from lower functions (1979). The crucial difference between them is that lower-order, "natural" mental functions are manifested in behaviors that are instinctive, reflexive, or *immediate*, whereas higher-order, "artificial," or "cultural" mental functions are realized in *mediated* activity. These latter constitute mental *tools*. Loosely analogous to the technical tools with which we organize, manipulate, and transform the physical world, our mental tools provide interpretive guidelines for structuring experience and understanding ourselves (Holland & Valsiner, 1988). They include signs, symbols, and systems of meaning that we use to "master" and interpret our own actions in relation to objects and persons in the environment. In kind, they range from relatively simple and intentionally deployed mnemonic strategies, such as tying a knot in a handkerchief, to the complex and deeply rooted myths and grand narratives with which we explain the cosmos and our origin and place within it.

That handkerchiefs, myths, narratives, even cabbages, become significant or meaningful through the constructive activities of the organism is a way of acknowledging such activity as a source of innovation, creativity, and novelty. For Paul Ricoeur (1972, 1976, 1983), the issue of social and cultural creativity is at the forefront of his investigations into narrative and hermeneutic practices. Telling stories, he argues, is the most permanent act of societies because it is the primary mode of recreating culture and thereby ensuring continuity through time (interview cited in Kerney, 1988). But culture and tradition can only pass itself on by fostering creative innovation. Jerome Bruner (1987) presses the same essential point in his highly successful effort to germinate narrative theory within developmental psychology. He argues that life amounts to the autobiography constructed:

> The heart of my argument is this: eventually the culturally shaped cognitive and linguistic processes that guide the self-telling of life narratives achieve the power to structure perceptual experience, to organize memory, to segment and purpose-build the very "events" of a life. In the end, we *become* the autobiographical narratives by which we "tell about" our lives. And given the cultural shaping to which I referred, we also become variants of the culture's canonical forms. I cannot imagine a more important psychological research project than one that addresses itself to the "development of autobiography"—how our way of telling about ourselves changes, and how these accounts come to take control of our ways of life. (p. 15; original italics)

It is apparent that as texts are penned, persons are created. And because our acts of self-invention are interpretive feats, because they are narrative achievements, they are necessarily drenched in cultural convention and practice; it is from this that they draw their communicative significance. The public and intersubjective nature of all meaning disqualifies any effort to identify interpretive activity with subjective intentions (Geertz, 1973). As Hermann Hesse insists, "If we were not something more than unique human beings . . . storytelling would lose all purpose" (1926/1968, p. 3). Vygotsky (1987) describes the creative process, both artistic and intellectual, as one in which inner, personal senses unfold their meanings as symbols-for-others. That is, meaning obtains only as a generalized concept, as an exteriorized social "fact." Locating narrative activity in social practice brings to the surface another reason why developmental psychologists have been eager to grapple with the interpretive paradigm: It resonates with their interests in linking human development to semiotic processes. There is now a broad-based movement to define personal identity as a beyond-the-skin "outreaching identity," and to bring a dialogical conception to the development of thinking and knowing (e.g., Rommetveit, 1991; Wertsch, 1991). Even moments of solitary meditation have been viewed as a sort of dialogue, an appeal from a momentary self to a better-considered self of the future (Peirce, 1977).

The assumption that human knowledge is mediated by signs and symbols constitutes the diadem of modern sociogenetic theory. Thus, Werner and Kaplan (1984) write that "in order to build up a truly human universe, that is, a world that is known rather than merely reacted to, man requires a new tool—an instrumentality that is suited for, and enables the realization of, those operations consti- tuting the activity of knowing" (p. 13). The idea was not at all for- eign to the progenitors of developmental psychology. James Mark Baldwin (1906) claims that it is only through social life that we be- come relatively separate, relatively private and thoughtful selves; Vy- gotsky (1979) argues a similar point in proposing that the higher functions of thought first appear in the collective life of children in the form of argumentation and only later develop into reflection for the individual child; Piaget, as well, believes that reflection can be viewed as internal argumentation—"the adult thinks socially, even when he is alone" (1955, p. 60).

Nevertheless, semiotic or dialogical mediation has only recent- ly gained wide attention as foundational to human development, and owes much of its current momentum to the popularity of Vy- gotsky's work. The centerpiece of his theory is that, as is true for our technical tools, semiotic processes provide the means by which we organize the world and make it meaningful. It is with them and through them that we manifest some measure of autonomy (reflec- tive awareness) from what we would otherwise "merely react to," and with this autonomy comes increased agency, planfulness, and control. These processes, language in particular, embody not only thought, but the history of human consciousness:

> [T]hinking and speech are the key to understanding the nature of hu- man consciousness. If language is as ancient as consciousness itself, if

language is consciousness that exists in practice for other people and therefore for myself, then it is not only the development of thought but the development of consciousness as a whole that is connected with the development of the word. . . . The word is the most direct manifestation of the historical nature of human consciousness. . . . The meaningful word is a microcosm of human consciousness. (Vygotsky, 1987, p. 285)

Extending the "word" to interpretive activity broadly conceived (see also Wertsch, 1985), we may say, therefore, that human development is not only a process of *construction* (and all that it entails vis-à-vis an active organism generating creative and innovative solutions to problems of adaptation), but is more properly described as a process of *semiotic* construction, of sign, narrative, text construction. Kenneth Burke (1966) reaches a similar conclusion in his understanding of humanity's "second nature." This consists of a complex network of symbolic systems—language, mathematics, music, dance, architectural styles, and so forth—with which we achieve a higher-order reflective awareness and thereby separate ourselves from our "natural condition" of appetitive desire.

The glint of evolutionary and historical implication calls attention to the third reason why genetic psychology is so well placed within the folds of the interpretive perspective—there is shared concern with the temporal organization of human knowledge. Piaget's very first sentence in *The Child and Reality* (1972) reads, "Child development is a temporal operation par excellence." When time is understood to reside in cultural and psychological structures, when it is understood to be both collected in the present and a canalizer of the future, it becomes also a conduit between past adaptations, habits, and traditions, and future innovation, invention, and creativity. Given this significance, it is not surprising that developmental and historical mechanisms are located there. Again, from *The Child and Reality*, Piaget writes:

The fact is that a discovery, a new notion, a statement, etc., must balance with the others. A whole play of regulation and of compensation is required to result in a coherence. I take the word *equilibrium* not in a static sense but in that of a progressive equilibration, the equilibrium being the compensation by reaction of the child to the outer disturbances, a compensation which leads to the operatory reversibility at the end of this development. Equilibrium appears to me to be the fundamental factor of this development. We then understand both the possibility of acceleration and at the same time the impossibility of an increase going beyond certain limits. (p. 29)

It seems banal to argue that there is no development or history in the absence of time, and no good theory of development or history that fails to take account of it. But some of the most influential historical figures in the discipline devoted considerable attention to making exactly this point.

SUBJECT AND OBJECT

Contemplating human knowledge and development as interpretive activity opens a window onto what many consider a solution to a classical problem—the relationship between the canonical and the personal, cultural and individual, objective and subjective. The exclusive Cartesian divide between the terms of each pair has haunted science for centuries. Yet however easy the modern consensus that a radical subject–object split can have only calamitous consequences (see Overton, 1994; Valsiner, 1987, 1994a; Wertsch, 1993), scholars have been slow to deliver coherent alternatives. Instead we have two equally worn and wounded paradigms with which to manage social science theory and methodology. One elevates the objective, and explains persons, as well as their knowledge, attitudes, experiences, and motivations, as outcomes of encounters with a mind-independent material reality (behaviorism). The other reverses the arrow of influence, elevates the subjective, and explains objective reality as the outcome of subjective mental processes (cognitivism).

On the face of it, the two are antithetical. However, they both emerged from a place where subject and object were construed as independent entities—the seedbed of 17th-century naturalism. Here the desire to enclose humankind within nature's circle was satisfied by abnegating self, agency, and consciousness (Taylor, 1985). This was the ground where objectivism was cultivated initially, but then suppressed as something overgrown and undesirable. Rooted in its very opposition, subjectivism flourished.

The kinship between subjectivism and objectivism is apparent in the way they both cleave to the machine categories of additive elementarism, linearity, and unidirectional causality (Overton, 1994; Valisner, 1987). Overton (1994) describes the self-sustaining struggle as one that is inherent to all dualisms:

> It is the nature of any split dualism that the failure of one of its terms necessarily supports the viability of the opposed term. Dualism references distinct entities and the manner in which these entities are joined. When dualism operates with "one term suppressed" the claim is made that the non-suppressed term, in this case the objective, will be the foundation for, and hence provide the account of, the suppressed term, the subjective. The objective is selected as The Real and it is to account for the subjective which is chosen as The Appearance. However, because it is a dualism, when the project begins to fail, the weight of evidence begins to shift to the suppressed term. Then the subjective becomes The Real and accounts for the objective. (p. 8)

It strikes me as somewhat remarkable that this same split frame has been used to impose a qualitative distinction between Piagetian and Vygotskian theories. Piagetian theory, with its outwardly cognitive and constructivist, cabbage-to-rabbit stance, has suffered complaints against its subjectivism, and accusations that it leaves no room for formative sociocultural processes and the network of institutions, beliefs, symbols, and ceremonies into which individuals are thrust. Vygotskian theory, very often touted as a panacea, struggles in turn against the pull of objectivism, and criticisms that it has the child so irretrievably embedded in social processes that it becomes impossible to extricate anything resembling an intact individual.

All of this goes to the point of how doggedly the subject–object dualism (here revealed as a cognitive–social dualism) pursues developmental theorizing. It has been noted, in fact, that the "cognitive revolution"—meant to remedy the ills of behaviorist doctrine by reacquainting psychology with such notions as "mind," "self," and "intentionality"—eventually took its form from the same mechanistic cast (Overton, 1994; Valsiner, 1991). A similar state of affairs obtains in the recent and widespread adoption of Vygotsky's theory by North American psychologists, which also may be characterized as a revolution, a "social" one, intended to unseat cognitivism. But within the subject–object dualism, a swing of the pendulum means only that we are once again seeking material causes for the emergence of psychological phenomena. This version of Vygotsky's sociogenetic theory is seen in a rash of studies that provide increasingly detailed descriptions of how local problem solutions are transferred over time from child plus others to child alone. Staying close to the paradigm of empirical–analytic psychology, and employing its traditional tools and methods, the overarching aim is to demonstrate causal connections between interpersonal interaction at Time 1 and intrapsychological functioning at Time 2. This is little more than retro-behaviorism.

The interpretive perspective, on the other hand, negotiates the boundary between subjective and objective by locating both within a relational field. Private and public, personal and canonical, individual and environment—these are not understood to be separate and independent entities, but mutually constituting features of an organized and unified system. This solution to the subject–object conundrum neither reduces one to the other nor denies the distinction between them—they constitute a unity, not an identity. In this regard, the interpretive paradigm may be yoked conceptually to the expressivist enterprise launched by 18th-century Romantics in opposition to the naturalism that preceded it. Naturalism, and its modern variants, presumes that knowledge resides in the degree of correspondence between subject and object (as in the amount or accuracy of "representations"), or in the efficiency with which correspondence is achieved. Romanticism, in contrast, views knowledge and most other mental phenomena as creative expression. Expression realizes and constitutes thought, memory, attention, emotion. Persons manifest their identities, and their reflective awareness, through the medium of expression.

Using the example of language as but one instance of expressive activity, Taylor (1985) provides an illustration by considering what it means to have a particular word, for example, "triangle," in one's lexicon. It means, certainly, that one can focus on the property of *shape*, rather than color, size, or smell; and it means that one can identify a *particular shape* as triangular, as opposed to oval or square. But what is remarkable is the understanding that "triangle" is the right and proper description of the object. This implication is the heart and soul of what it means to use language. It is to recognize triangles in the "strong sense," and not merely react to them; it is to be conscious of them in a "fuller way," to be more reflectively aware.

The expressive doctrine is a significant departure from naturalism and its empiricist offspring. Its connection with reflective awareness, Taylor (1985) argues, opens a new dimension:

> If language serves to express/realize a new kind of awareness; then it may not only make possible a new awareness of things, an ability to describe them; but also new ways of feeling, of responding to things. . . . The revolutionary idea of expressivism was that the development of new modes of expression enables us to have new feelings, more powerful or more refined, and certainly more self-aware. In being able to express our feelings, we give them a reflective dimension which transforms them. . . . From this perspective, we cannot draw a boundary around the language of prose in the narrow sense, and divide it off from those other symbolic–expressive creations of man: poetry, music, art, dance, etc. (pp. 232–233)

INTERPRETIVE STANCES IN DEVELOPMENTAL PSYCHOLOGY

Given the common ground of interpretive and organismic approaches surveyed above, it comes as no surprise that the history of genetic psychology can be read as a chronicle of similar arguments. Vygotsky's writings abound with criticism for methods that treat the environment as isolated from the child, rather than in terms of "what it means for the child":

> We have inadequately studied the internal relationship of the child to the people around him. . . . We have recognized in words that we need to study the child's personality and environment as a unity. It is incorrect, however, to represent this problem in such a way that on one side we have the influence of the personality while on the other we have the influence of the environment. Though the problem is frequently represented in precisely this way, it is incorrect to represent the two as external forces acting on one another. In the attempt to study the unity, the two are initially torn apart. The attempt is then made to unite them. (translated in Minick, 1987, p. 32)

Vygotsky's solution was to define "experience" as the basic unit that manifests the child's internal relationship with its environment. It constitutes the "unit of personality and environment as they exist in development." Kurt Lewin (1933) employed similar rhetoric in discussing the dynamic unity of child and environment and attempting to define methodologically the "real environments" of children, as opposed to the "objective" physical or social environments as seen through the eyes of others. Piaget expressed similar sentiments: "the social fact for us is a fact to be explained, not to be invoked as an extra-psychological factor" (1962, p. 4).

These ideas have been revived and modernized by a number of scholars concerned with issues of human development and culture. For example, Bruner's narrative perspective addresses the problem of characterizing boundaries between the personal and canonical. Bruner (1987, 1990) argues that life narratives, and the persons who create and become them, must cohere with a "community of life stories." Community implies, in fact, some "deep structure" of connection and shared understanding between listeners and tellers. Believing that the success of the cognitive revolution in psychology has resulted in a technocratic fragmentation of the "person," he holds out some hope that a more interpretive, narrative perspective will reintegrate individuals into cultural structures and restore some semblance of personal unity:

> This conviction is based on two connected arguments. The first is that to understand man you must understand how his experiences and his acts are shaped by his intentional states, and the second is that the form of these intentional states is realized only through participation in the symbolic systems of the culture. Indeed, the very shape of our lives—the rough and perpetually changing draft of our autobiography that we carry in our minds—is understandable to ourselves and to others only by virtue of those cultural systems of intepretation. But culture is also constitutive of mind. By virtue of this actualization in culture, meaning achieves a form that is public and communal rather than private and autistic. Only by replacing this transactional model of mind with an isolating, individualistic one have Anglo-American philosophers been able to make Other Minds so opaque and impenetrable. (pp. 33–34)

Throughout his recent work on narrative, Bruner presses the point that all human action has multiple interpretive levels. This general proposition has been used to great advantage in exploring children's development in cultural context. Jean Briggs's (1992) recent study of Inuit children's play is an especially thorough example of a methodology through which multiple interpretations may be seen to cohere into dramatic structures. Karen Ann Watson-Gegeo (1992) likewise makes a case for and presents a form of "thick interpretation" in her study of school failure among children from third-world communities.

Eschewing the volume of research that construes the child–culture relationship in terms of dependent and independent variables, and uniformly dissatisfied with both the active child–passive environment ontology of cognitivism, and the passive child–active environment ontology of behaviorism, a growing number of developmentalists argue that owing to our belief in the inevitable progress of empirical science, our unquestioning adherence to statistical methodology, and our abiding trust in the ultimate truth of common sense, developmental psychology has lost its epistemological moorings and is in need of a radical reconstruction. Those expressing such rogue sentiments are concerned to characterize the interdependence of two dynamic processes: the development of children and the development of the cultural contexts in which they live. Both are structured, both are active, and both require formal analysis if we are to make headway in knowing "how the child's encounter with the external world becomes functional in bringing new psychological functions into being" (Valsiner & van der Veer, 1993, p. 58).

And what is the nature of the child's encounter with the world? This question is a pedal point of tension for nearly all sociogenetic theories because a large part of what it means to be "sociogenetic" is to hold to the position that it is the *encounter* that precipitates development (e.g., Rogoff, 1990; Wertsch, 1985). Valsiner's (1987) "individual–sociological" theoretical framework is a noteworthy example. From his perspective, children's thoughts and actions are understood to emerge from transactions with an environment at least partially defined by the intentional actions of others. On this reading, his point of departure differs hardly at all from those of other sociogenetic theorists, all of whom pledge to what Harré

(1991) has labeled the *sociality thesis*: "All action meaningful as acts, that is, action which is capable of sustaining some psychological phenomenon such as remembering or deciding, is joint action" (p. 155). But whereas the psychological activities of individuals—the intellectual and emotional processes that bear on their subjectivities, their personal and private desires, goals, fantasies, reminiscences, and world views—have been written out of many contemporary sociogenetic narratives, the interpretive perspective presented here insists on their centrality.

The reason for clinging so tenaciously to a formal analytical account of the subject is that to fail to do so is to collapse psychological development onto social contingency, which is to make incoherent the entire socio*genetic* enterprise. In other words, although we might yet hold to the sociality thesis, or what Valsiner and van der Veer (1988) name the "ontological postulate," that human cognition is inherently social in nature, we lose all sight of its implicative genetic counterpart, the "developmental postulate" that human cognition *becomes* social, indeed, becomes *cognitive*, by virtue of the subject acting in a sociocultural context.

Jaan Valsiner's concept of *inclusive separation* (1987, 1992, 1994a) is illuminating in this regard. It provides a semantic tool for recognizing that we are separate from our environments, although interdependent with them, and that the intersubjective world that we forge together by way of transcending our subjectivities, and to which we refer as "common" or "collective," is in fact only partially shared. This constitutes the very foundation of all metacommunicative process: In entering a dialogue or communicative exchange, the person acts "as if" meanings are common, "as if" the other is similarly oriented and like-minded, and the whole process of negotiating shared understanding is wrapped in personal reconstructions of "as if," of metaphor. So it is that negotiating meaning, constructing an intersubjective and partially shared reality, becomes the fountainhead of subjectivity—the source of its emergence and differentiation. Valsiner argues, moreover, that because the personal and the collective are dynamic, structured systems, and yoked in an interdependent and coevolutionary process,

> social-psychological (collective) and individual-psychological phenomena are of the same developmental origin—the former being the

result of *externalization* of previously existing "personal cultures" of participants in the social discourse, the latter the result of *internalization* of different aspects of the social discourse. As a result of internalization, the "personal culture" develops further as the organizer of the individual person's psychological life. The individual "personal culture" does not reflect the "collective culture" as its "mirror image"—since it is constructed and re-constructed by the person de novo in the context of social discourse. (1989, p. 507)

A major purpose of Valsiner's theoretical agenda, and one with special significance for understanding adolescent risk-taking, is to elevate the status of novelty as a salient feature of ontogeny and cultural history. He argues, quite reasonably, I think, that if we do not at some level address the coming-into-existence of things that are entirely new (to paraphrase Lorenz, 1972), then we do not address development. Apparently, during medieval ages the instrument of emergent novelty was thought to be *fulguration*: nothing less than God's own lightening. Although it seems too often true that in our modern age only the words have changed—that is, upon closer scrutiny terms like "internalization," "appropriation," and "equilibration" seem more magic than science (Winegar, in press)—we are nonetheless on the lookout for instruments of a more earthly and empirical origin.

Although the corpus of Valsiner's work shows an early and abiding interest in the problem of emergent novelty, his most recent efforts have been directed toward situating development in irreversible time (1992, 1994b). He quotes Prigogine with enthusiasm: "The renewal of science is to a large extent the history of the rediscovery of time" (cited in Valsiner, 1992, p. 35). Seeing in this rediscovery some hope for addressing certain of our major theoretical conundrums, central among them the coordination of relations between different temporal levels of analysis (i.e., phylogenesis, ontogenesis, microgenesis, and cultural history; see also Cole, 1992; Gariépy, 1995), Valsiner attempts to overcome the spatial metaphors to which our understanding of development cleaves so easily. Internal–external, subjective–objective, personal–cultural: These dualities take on new meaning when located in time rather than space. In particular, they permit a view of development as "constructive adaptation" through which new internal/subjective/personal organization forms emerge as anticipations of external/objective/cultural possibilities—of what might be, rather than what is. This can be extended to a view of the child who reaches "as if" objects can be grasped; speaks or plays "as if" meanings can be shared. And so they are. The "feed-forward" quality of child action—its role as a mechanism of preadaptation—speaks to the child's contribution to its own developmental future. Thus, the child canalizes its environment just as the intentional actions of others canalize child action. Both are dynamic, structured, interdependent systems, and the "goodness of their misfit" (Valsiner & Cairns, 1992) guarantees their continuing coevolution.

And what of risk-taking? "Uncertainty," writes Lopes (1993), "is embedded in time. There is a now in which some things are true, a future in which other things may be true, and a still farther future in which we may reflect on the past. At the point of choice we look forward along this track, and we also anticipate looking back. The temporal element is what gives risk both savor and sting" (p. 289)

THE MERELY KNOWN AND THE IMAGINATIVELY KNOWN

Metaphorical and imaginative processes have become targets for analysis in interpretive theory. They are thought, in particular, to organize the structure of knowledge and experience. For Ricoeur, "imagination" provides a solution to one of the most crucial problems confronting hermeneutics: the relation between tradition and innovation. The hermeneutic imagination operates in a double capacity that binds tradition and innovation within a relationship of complementarity rather than antagonism: "Insofar as it secures the function of recollecting and reiterating types across discontinuous episodes, imagination is plainly on the side of tradition. And insofar as it fulfills its equally essential function of projecting new horizons of possibility, imagination is committed to the role of semantic—and indeed ontological—innovation" (interview cited in Kerney, 1988, p. 24).

Ricoeur understands the function of tradition to be analogous to our grand paradigmatic narrative forms; they provide the grammar that directs the composition of new works, but are incapable of eradicating the creative role of poiesis that makes each work unique and original. Tradition and creative innovation are thus conjoined within the singular process of imagination.

Overton (1994) plays out a similar theme in describing "metaphor" as an interpretive process that structures the "phenomenological matrix." It includes two recursively joined spheres of influence—the sphere of imaginative processes and the sphere of inferential processes:

> The sphere of imagination is activity that launches metaphor from the familiar realm—regardless of whether familiar is defined as sensory–motor activity scheme or linguistic expression. The sphere of inferential is activity that structures the unfamiliar in terms of the familiar and thus gives shape and meaning to inquiry. Metaphor as a process then operates projectively beginning from the known, giving meaning to the unknown, and recursively resulting in a restructuring of the known. Interpretive activity moves from imagination to inference to imagination. (p. 219)

Nourished by paradigms and metaphors once considered the province of literary and aesthetic traditions, those interested in human development and culture are developing a persuasive rhetoric, if not yet a formal language, that includes "cultural genres," "texts of identity," and "the storied nature of human conduct." They are wrestling with issues of creativity, imagination, drama, experiment. Perhaps James Mark Baldwin's neglected third volume of *Thought and Things* (1911), focused as it is on interest and art, will gain some currency in this changing climate. He argues there that cognition consists of two mutually dependent factors:

> Every such object (secured by consciousness) is either one of *knowledge*, recognized as part of the actual, the external, the true; or is one of *assumption*, "*semblance*," or *make-believe*, one to be toyed with, "sembled" or *Eingefuhlt*, one to get satisfaction from, to image for personal purposes and selective handling, with some measure of disregard of its exact place and relations in the sphere of the actual. The *actual* and the *imaginative*, the merely known and the usefully or playfully or aesthetically—in short the semblantly or imaginatively—known, *is the*

universal and ever-present contrast in the meanings of cognition. (p. 4; original italics)

With uncanny resemblance to modern interpretive approaches, Baldwin claims that every cognitive content, every "thing" apprehended by consciousness, must have both renderings. Moreover, "the mergings and reversals of one into the other turn out to show the very nerve of the process of development of knowledge" (p. 5). But whereas the "actualizing" mode is comprised of commonly shared, relatively static, presupposed, and "truthful" meanings, the "imaginative" mode constitutes the dynamic factor that is instrumental to those meanings. In other words, general systems of meaning follow in the wake of ludic and aesthetic constructions, yet also chart a course for future constructions: *Belief motives make-believe and make-believe engenders belief:*

> What is instrumental is not truth; but the imagination of something that may become truth. . . . Not only is all truth due to the imagination, having been in the first place experimentally entertained and then confirmed; it is always in a process of flux and flow. And this gives it its main value; for thus it assumes continually its role of feeding the imagination for further discovery of fact and further control by the self. The mere telling over of actualities, the items of true and accomplished judgment, is hardly worthwhile, save possibly to the intellectual miser who loves the mere glint of his erudition; on the contrary, the real thinker is he who melts the known in the crucible of hypothesis, of imaginative speculation, and draws out new casts for common circulation. (Baldwin, 1911, p. 8)

I hope this brief excursion through the history of ideas brings us close enough to the center of things to appreciate the cultural–historical implications of the interpretive turn, and its seductions for genetic psychology. Within its broad, multidisciplinary sweep, we are moving with fresh but familiar language and insight toward an understanding of human development and culture as a process of construction that is semiotically mediated and temporally organized. We are urged to consider the nature of knowledge as something prospective, experimental, and playful, and thereby to locate the source of reflective awareness, agency, and formative experience.

THE EVOLUTION OF SELF AND CONCEPTIONS
OF TRANSFORMATIVE EXPERIENCE

With the heroes, man takes his first step beyond the necessary,
into the realm of risk, defiance, shrewdness, deceit, art.
—ROBERTO CALASSO

Surveying a vast landscape of philosophy, literature, and science, it cannot be far from true to say that the evolution of self during adolescence has drawn more attention than any other aspect of children's development. It is during adolescence that childhood identities are remade in vital ways. The adolescent touches for the first time an inner space, an inward self. And for the first time, imagination and fantasy are turned toward the "intimate realm" of experience to express inner desires, motives, impulses, and attractions (Vygotsky, 1994; aslo see Lightfoot, in press-a). Created here are individuals who pursue a greater depth of intimacy in relationships, who stride toward their own agency, individuation, and mastery of circumstance; and who are capable of acting with higher levels of compassion and the authority of moral conviction. Such developments bear on the changing relationship between persons and the worlds they live in. Viewed as a temporal process, be it the development of an individual self, or the historical evolution of cultural conceptions of self, it becomes clear that this relationship has constituted persons as individuals, worlds as dynamic contexts of action, and risks as transformative experience.

It has been noted that at some flash point in the history of human understanding, people became individuals. A curious observation on the face of it. What was a man before that? had he not eyes? had he not hands, organs, dimensions, senses, affections, passions? He was fed with the same food, hurt with the same weapons, warmed and cooled by the same winter and summer. Thus did Lionel Trilling (1971, pp. 24–25) summon Shylock to make the point that although it was once enough to claim membership in the human race by giving account of the body's parts, functions, and brute reactions, there are certain things a man did not have or do until he became an individual. When people became individuals, they acquired a hitherto unknown awareness of internal space, a capacity to imagine themselves in multiple roles and to regard themselves from other points of view; they acquired, as well, some sense of audience, a public over and against which to construct a private, agentic, and autonomous "I."

Modern conceptions of self manifest centuries of human cultural evolution. Renaissance thought of the 15th and 16th centuries marks a mutation between the theological belief system of the Middle Ages, and a scientific interpretation of reality that came of age during the Enlightenment period. It was here that "world" and "man" were discovered: The Copernican revolution restructured our fundamental understanding of the world's position in the universe; the Reformation restructured our fundamental understanding of man's position in the world. These changes penetrated the core of basic assumptions concerning the very nature of reality—of space, time, and consciousness. Bakhtin (1986) explains that as the earth's solar system and its relations to other worlds were determined,

> it became subject to interpretation and, in a real-life sense, historical. It is not just a matter of the quantity of great discoveries, new journeys, and acquired knowledge, but rather of that new *quality* in the comprehension of the real world that results from all this: from being a fact of abstract consciousness, theoretical constructs, and *rare books*, the new *real* unity and integrity of the world became a fact of ordinary books and everyday thoughts. (p. 44; original italitcs)

Subject to interpretation. Historical. These are telling words. And by what fairy magic has the world become really real? How has a concrete and ordinary world been constructed out of the abstract and theoretical? These developments, in fact, prophecy a subject who construes the world-as-object, who holds it at such a distance that it becomes a "psychological possession" (Winnicott, 1971), capable of being examined, known, and experienced more directly.

As the world is made object, so too is the self. Literature provides a historical record of transformations to what Rorty (1976) describes as the "entities we have invented ourselves to be." It is important to know this record, to stay on nodding terms with those former selves who inhabit and define the literary canon, because doing so lends clarity to our personal constructions (see also Bruner, 1987) and the way we understand *experience* to enter and shape our lives. I am interested in conceptions of experience, especially *forma-tive* experience, because, as we shall see, it is an issue that adolescents often dwell on in recounting and justifying their risk-taking activities. Stated in the broadest of terms, teenagers consider their risks to stand as declarations of identity, as badges of peer group membership, and seek risks actively for their capacity to challenge, educate, and restructure the status quo, be it the authority of parents, physical limits, social relationships, or feelings of confidence, competence, and responsibility. In other words, adolescents understand their risks to be avatars of the self—to provide a depth of experience that is at one and the same time personally and interpersonally demonstrative and transformative (see also Lightfoot, 1992).

The question of what makes for formative or transformative experience has recently engaged the attention of cultural anthropologists and psychologists, especially those of an interpretive ilk, who are looking for some dramatic substrate or emotional current capable of conveying life narratives, of keeping them satisfactory, worthwhile, interesting, moving, and, in a real sense, livable (Abrahams, 1986; Sarbin, 1990). Crites (1986) goes so far as to recommend that we reserve the word "experience" for what is incorporated into one's story, and "thus owned, owned up to, appropriated" (p. 161). Scheibe (1986) expresses a similar sentiment in reflecting on dramatic experience as essential experience: "In terms of psychological biography, a life lived on a single plane is simply insufficient as a story—it doesn't go anywhere, it doesn't move. The socius is constantly testing the individual for the satisfactoriness of the unfolding narrative, and the particular socius in which we are immersed wants change, wants variation, wants dramatic build and decline" (p. 133).

An etymology of *experience* reveals that the affinities between risk and experience are deeply rooted. Etymologically, *experience* is derivative of the Indo-European base *per*, meaning to "attempt, venture, risk," and, as in *experiment*, "to try or test." Its link to risk-taking is revealed more fully in its suffixed, extended form *peri-tlo*, meaning "trial, danger, peril." Reaching deeper, we find meanings associated with moving forward in time. The Greek verb *perao* means "I pass through." Pulling these various senses together, we have what Victor Turner described as a "laminated semantic system focused on *experience*, which portrays it as a journey, as a test (of self, of suppositions about others), a ritual passage, an exposure to peril or risk, a source of fear" (1982, pp. 17–18). Turner laminated yet another sense onto these ancient meanings by embedding them within Wilhelm Dilthey's and John Dewey's social philosophies, each of which sought to identify distinctive units of experience separate from "mere experience" for the purpose of gaining insight into the aesthetics of everyday life. By both accounts, life is more intense, vital, and meaningful during moments of passage between disturbance and harmony. As William James argues, "Life is in the transitions as much as the terms connected. Often, indeed, it seems to be there more emphatically, as if our spurts and sallies forward were the real living line of the battle . . ." (in McDermott, 1967, p. 212).

Stephen Lyng's (1993) concept of risk-taking as "edgework" is relevant in this context. Pulling at the common thread holding together activities as diverse as skydiving, drug abuse, and entrepreneurial business, Lyng argues that all may be properly subsumed under the concept of "boundary negotiation." The concept is intended to capture the efforts of individuals to define limits and explore boundaries between life and death, consciousness and unconsciousness, illness and well-being, or "any other dramatic experiential expression of the line between order and disorder" (p. 110).

All of these ideas converge on the belief that life is *lived* through trial, risk, and adventure; that it takes its form from the experiences that fill it; that it is, as Hellen Keller writes, a "daring adventure, or nothing." Risks are set clearly apart from the ongoing flow of experience because they are novel, and it is their experimental nature—the fact that the individual who has them or seeks them leaves terra firma to do so—that affords them special status, and makes for vivid experience. Indeed, the entire enterprise of adolescent risk-taking is quixotic, a struggle for something just out of reach.

Nonetheless, the idea that daring adventure is the stuff of ordinary lives lived by ordinary people, and that experience of this particular sort can shape people's lives, or by marking a leading edge, suggest some life-course trajectory, has emerged only recently in cultural history, and I suspect that it doesn't make its ontogenetic debut until adolescence. The interview material indicates that this idea can be articulated fairly well by many 16- to 18-year-olds. This is no mere coincidence. The personal is cognate with the canonical, and these recursive iterations of form constitute hard evidence that both are driven by the same interpretive processes. By examining the evolution of the hero in literature, we will throw light on the ontogeny of self-as-seeker-of-experience. Two developments will become relevant to an emerging conception of experience as transformative: One is the differentiation and integration of self and world (or subject and object, more generally); the other is an increasing and deeper infusion of historical and biographical time. Conjoined, these two developments permit the introduction of *depth* into experience itself.

LITERARY FORMS OF THE HERO

In her analysis of the written record from ancient to modern times, Rorty (1976) identifies five literary *types*. The first one is manifested in Greek "characters," whose fate, choices, and actions, however noble or tragic, devolve directly from their parentage. Biblical and sacred "figures" emerge later; they lead exemplary lives, but are neither formed by nor own their experiences. "Persons" arrive on the literary scene when it becomes more fully dramatic. They *choose* their roles, and as agents of their own actions and destinies, are held responsible and accountable for them. They suffer crises of identity, question their own moral integrity, and insist on "freedom" and "autonomy" within which to make their choices. Rorty continues her analysis through the evolution of "selves," and finally "individuals" each entity distinguished from its predecessor by virtue of increased agency, individuation, self-consciousness, and ownership of experience.

The historical parade of characters, figures, persons, selves, and individuals shows a gradual differentiation and integration of self and world. As selves become more individuated and reflectively aware, more connected with themselves, they also become increasingly embedded in reality. This lately arriving connection between self and world admits the possibility of mutual transformation, that one might effectively press upon the other, and makes room for construing persons and their worlds in terms of biographical and historical processes.

These ideas carried Bakhtin (1986) through a historical analysis of the novel as a literary genre. The infusion of temporal processes culminates in the *Bildungsroman*, a form of the novel that details the psychological development of the principal character. Bakhtin finds a prototype in Goethe's notion of the *fullness of time*, set forth as a counterpoint to the tendency of contemporary romantics to idealize the past by cutting it away from the "unbroken line of development." The past must be understood as "creatively effective," with impact on the present, and clearing a path for the "necessary future." This constitutes the *fullness of time*, a "graphic, visible completeness" of reality and the people who constitute it: "Everything is visible, everything is concrete, everything is corporeal, and everything is material in this world, and at the same time everything is intensive, interpreted, and creatively necessary" (Bakhtin, 1986, p. 43). Ortega y Gasset (1914/1961) moves in the same direction in his description of the epic and the mythical past that occupies it. It is not a remembered past, but rather an ideal yesterday that eludes recollection or identification with the present. The epic is about another world in another time, cut off entirely from the cord of history that defines *our* past and that we can imagine as being a once-present reality.

According to Bakhtin, as time enters literature, it provides a more integrated picture of the world and life, and thus becomes more "profoundly realistic." The capacity to present "real-life whole" is the source of artistic significance. But the reality, the real-life that accompanies the infusion of time, is not that of a material world as conceived by those who view subject and object in dualistic terms. Bakhtin exerts considerable effort dispelling any such notion. He vilifies the realism of the 18th-century Enlightenment, which established empiricism as the only legitimate path to knowledge and in doing so impoverished the world by narrowing what constitutes the real:

> Much in the world turns out to be unreal, illusory, and it is cast out as prejudice, fantasy, or fabrication; the world turns out to be more impoverished than it had seemed to others in past ages or to the hero himself in his youth. Many of the hero's illusions about himself are dispelled, and he becomes more serious, drier, and more impoverished. Such unification of the world and man is typical of the critical and abstract realism of the Age of the Enlightenment. (1986, cited by editors in footnote, p. 58)

Thus, the realism construed here is not a literal or material realism, but a realism of interpretation: "[Anything that can be understood] always exists among other meanings as a link in the chain of meaning, which in its totality is the only thing that can be real" (Bakhtin, 1986, cited in editors' introduction; also see Overton, 1991, for a discussion of the different meanings of "realism" in psychology).

Several novelistic forms anticipate Goethe's vision. Bakhtin identifies each according to the confluence of hero, world, plot type, and composition—all mutually determining constituents. We can remain true to his conclusions, and stay closer to the task at hand, by focusing on images of the relation between the hero and the world. We will see that as time is introduced into the novel, the hero is considered to *develop*, the world becomes historical, and the relation between them becomes *experiential*—defines, in fact, what it means to experience.

One of the earliest forms is the *travel novel*. The hero is undistinguished here, occupies little artistic attention, and serves mainly as a pointer that the novelist moves from one location to another to illustrate the world's diversity. It is a diversity of particulars, however, of countries, cultures, and nationalities whose differences and contrasts are those of simple spatial location. The hero, positioned in the north, speaks of northern things; positioned in the south, he speaks of different, southern things. Life itself is ordered by simple contrasts: happiness–unhappiness, success–failure, victory–defeat. Apuleius's *Metamorphoses*, known also as *The Golden Ass*, demonstrates this extraordinarily well as the only surviving Latin novel. In this story, the narrator swallows a potion, hoping to become an owl, but something goes awry and he becomes instead an ass. Despite the title, Apuleius devotes scant attention to this remarkable transformation, focusing instead on the ass's travels through Greece as he passes from one master to another. The transformation itself matters hardly at all, and provides little more than an excuse to move from place to place so as to provide a firsthand account of the world's vast variety.

The stability of world and hero, as Bakhtin describes it, is due to the underdeveloped conception of *time*. In concert with the emphasis on contrasts and particulars, the only significant temporal category is adventure time, which consists of "the most immediate units—moments, hours, days—snatched at random from the temporal process" (1986, p. 11). Historical time, absent in the travel novel, could provide an intrinsic tie that binds nations, countries, and social groups, but without it these sociocultural phenomena, even in their diversity, are no more than a colorful mosaic of steady juxtapositions between the familiar and the exotic. Likewise for the central character: the absence of "biological time" yields a hero who changes location but never point of view. "This novel," writes Bakhtin, "does not recognize human emergence and development. Even if his status changes sharply (in the picaresque novel he changes from beggar to rich man, from homeless wanderer to nobleman), he himself remains unchanged" (1986, p. 11).

A second early novelistic form, and the logical counterpart to the first, is the *novel of ordeal*. It was contemporaneous with the travel novel, and considerably more common. Whereas the world was the foreground of the travel novel, the hero takes center stage in the novel of ordeal. Bakhtin defines several subcategories (including the Greek romance, medieval chivalric, and baroque forms), but they all depict the world as an arena for testing an idealized, complete, and unchanging hero. The hero may be tested for valor, strength, fidelity, or faith, but the tests "do not become formative experience for him, they do not change him, and in that very immutability of the hero lies the entire point" (1986, p. 13). The point, of course, is that the hero arrives on the scene in prefabricated perfection. Predictably, he springs forward fully formed, as did Athena from the head of Zeus and Aphrodite from the foam of the sea. Gilgamesh is another example. His story survives precariously in scraps of lore and broken tablets that predate Homeric epic by one and a half thousand years (Sandars, 1960). He is our most ancient hero, and the gods saw to it that he was among the most marvelous: they made him two-thirds god and one-third man; they made him wise and showed him mysteries and secret things; they endowed him with courage and beauty. But like his heroic progeny, Gilgamesh remains untouched by worldly experience; he was the one who always knew; never the seeker or scholar.

In the same way that the hero remains untouched by worldly experience, the world remains unaffected by the efforts and actions of those within it. There is no interaction, in other words, between subject and object, between the hero and the world in which he must prove himself. Again Bakhtin (1986) points to the influence of time. Adventure time is more developed in the novel of ordeal because the plot is more developed. It is composed as a string of extraordinary occurrences that interrupt the typical sequence or timing of life's events. These occurrences lack any historical or biographical duration or significance. This is apparent in the manner by which they are inserted, as bounded and isolated episodes, between what *ought* to be contiguous moments of ordinary biography. In Greek romance, for example, something happens between betrothal and the wedding, or between the wedding and the wedding night. But once the hero overcomes the impediment, life returns to normal: The lovers marry; the marriage is consummated. This is not a matter of ordinary life skirting some obstacle and then wending back to the beaten path. Even this would exaggerate the reach of adventure into biographical time. Its isolation is so complete that it can only pause normal biography, which resumes its inevitable course as soon as the adventure runs out. Sandars says of Gilgamesh, who struggles admirably but unsuccessfully against his humanity, that his return home was "like the breaking of a spell, when at the end of trouble and search and with a prize almost won, everything suddenly returns to ordinary and we are back where we started" (1960, p. 43).

All of this begins to change during the 16th century, a time that ushered in the "age of adventure" and a qualitatively new image of the hero (Ortega y Gasset, 1914/1961; Schiebe, 1986). The historic leap is marked by Cervantes's *Don Quixote*, published in 1605/1615. Quixote is our first *romantic* hero because he is the first who desires to reform reality and dislocate the material order. Espousing his own realism of interpretation, Ortega argues that the real is not what is seen, but what is foreseen, and the role of adventure is to embrace the unforeseen, the un-thought-of, and the new. Scheibe seconds this notion in construing adventure as part of a dynamic movement between repose and novelty, between redundancy and change. To oscillate between them is to experience, and what distinguishes our fresh-faced hero from the one of former times is his *will* to experience, his *will* to adventure, his *aim* o alter the course of things and live beyond the ordinary and habitual. He is the first actually to *take* a risk, and he presents a new role for adventure in constructing biography.

The *biographical novel* itself is a third novelistic category, and it takes yet another step away from a radical subject–object dualism toward a dynamic duality and the experience, personal development, and historicity that such a duality implies. Although its predecessors include classical biographies, autobiographies, and Christian confessionals, these were but dim outlines for a category that was never to be fully formed because its position in literary history was usurped in the mid-1800s by the *Bildungsroman*. However, by the 18th century the biographical novel takes on some shape as a general principle for configuring the hero. First of all, the hero is de-heroized. He is portrayed with positive and negative characteristics; bad, perhaps, but in an endearing or roguish way. Such is Henry Fielding's introduction of Tom Jones: "As we determined, when we first sat down to write this history, to flatter no man, but to guide our pen throughout by the directions of truth, we are obliged to bring our hero on the stage in a much more disadvantageous manner than we could wish; and to declare honestly, even at his first appearance, that it was the universal opinion of all . . . that he was certainly born to be hanged" (Fielding, 1749/1963, p. 73).

In contrast to the splendid—and remote—Gilgamesh, Tom arrives on stage disheveled, with dirt under his nails and a stolen apple in his pocket. We know him well. The biographical novel is a significant departure from its predecessors because it draws in just this manner toward the typical and quotidian—everyone a hero, every life an adventure. Still, although world and hero now travel along a shared and mutually defined trajectory, there is no sense that either has the capacity to reconfigure the other in any essential or fundamental way. The life path depicted is paved with objective results (works, deeds, feats, and so forth), or the subjective feelings associated with them (happiness/unhappiness), which are no less material or inevitable for being internal. "The hero's life and fate change," writes Bakhtin, "they assume structure and evolve, but the hero himself remains essentially unchanged" (1986, p. 17).

It wasn't until the second half of the 18th century that literature provides an image of the hero as an individual-in-progress. The three novelistic categories—the travel novel, the novel of ordeal, and the biography—laid the groundwork for the synthetic *Bildungsroman* (the "novel of education") that emerged in Germany and portrays a hero in the process of becoming. For virtually all other novel forms, the hero is "a *constant* in the novel's formula and all other quantities—the spatial environment, social position, fortune, in brief, all aspects of the hero's life and destiny—can therefore be *variables*" (Bakhtin, 1986, p. 21). In contrast to the static unity of the ready-made hero, the central character of the *Bildungsroman* projects a dynamic unity whose changes acquire *plot* significance. As the hero becomes a variable, changes infect the interpretation or construction of the entire narrative. "Time is introduced into man, enters into his very image, changing in a fundamental way the significance of all aspects of his destiny and life." (p. 21)

In the *Bildungsroman*, concepts of time take on depth and complexity that are absent in other forms. Biographical time appears as *real* time—limited, unique, irreversible. It also participates in the larger and longer process of historical time. The world and the events that occupy it are no longer window dressing for showing the hero to his best advantage. Encounters between hero and world no longer suggest happenstance, but appear by design, or *of* design. Other characters, places, and objects take on meaning in the life of the hero. To use Bakhtin's language, they acquire a "life-determining essence." Adventures, also, are located in the more complex time of biography and history, and from here draw their significance and their reality. To wit, they have undergone a transformation similar to that of the de-heroized hero: They are no longer adventurous, at least in the classical sense of being demonstrations or exhibitions of the hero's ready-to-hand preparedness and aptitude. Situated in time, both hero and world experiences become "more profoundly realistic."

We have, finally, a fully modern hero who is understood to develop through time, and who has and is shaped by experience actively sought. Goethe's *fullness of time*, that unbroken line of development by which the past carves a direction for the necessary future, is what Bergson (1911; see also Valsiner, 1994c) means when he speaks of *creative evolution*, it is what Gould (1987) has in mind when he describes geological *deep time*, and it is what James Mark Baldwin (1911) refers to when he describes the imaginative, hypothetical, playful, aesthetic, and speculative mode of cognition as an instrument for apprehending reality. In the absence of real time, or full time, or deep time, experiences are cut away, and become historical clutter, detritus. In the absence of deep time, experience is decorative rather than formative, and persons not in possession of their experiences lack the depth and purpose these experiences provide and the interpersonal connection that comes from sharing them.

The introduction of deep time introduces a depth of experience denied by those web-like constructions that have become recently popular as metaphors of our lives—the social networks; neural nets; the Internet; the webs of knowledge, beliefs, desires—those vast and sprawling two-dimensional constructions in which many things are connected laterally, but nothing is touched deeply. The modern hero contrives to hold to some hierarchical scheme in order to distinguish the small from the grand, in order to vanquish minutiæ. In the face of nets and webs, the modern hero insists on some transcendental center that holds, is whole and perdurable. To be such a hero is to privilege the spider, to be one among many. Ultimately, and as Ortega insists, it is to be oneself.

CHAPTER 4

Play as
Interpretive Activity

Theories of play provide a scaffold for understanding the drama of adolescent social life as a form of interpretive activity that entrains culture in individuals, and contributes to the development of self as social participant. Perspectives from anthropology and developmental psychology will be explored, with special attention to those that resonate with a general interpretive perspective. Largely preoccupied with the constitution and transformation of self–culture relations, these perspectives present play as text, as story or narrative construction where meanings are inscribed and thereby made intelligible. This is especially apparent in the anthropological work, for example, Clifford Geertz's (1972), in which play is considered as a form of social commentary. Applied to the case of adolescent social life, risk-taking is conceptualized as "deep play"—a declaration of one's place in the social scheme of things, and a means of participating in peer group life. From a more psychological orientation, we will explore play as a vehicle of the imagination. D. W. Winnicott's (1971) insights into the aesthetics of everyday life, as well as Vygotsky's recently published writings on adolescent imagination and fantasy (in van der Veer & Valsiner, 1994), will help to make the case that the speculative, experimental, and future-oriented nature of adolescent risk-taking, like that of children's play and adults' literary and scientific works, constitutes and transforms relations between self and culture.

According to the research to be presented here, child and adult play has a mission: to illuminate self in relation to other. It campaigns for clarification. It aims to elucidate and comment upon what would otherwise be reflexive, spontaneous, arbitrary, unframed, overflowing, and unexamined. In the following pages we will see that this mission is spurred on two sides. One is a goading on behalf of epistemological concerns, the other on matters of socio-cultural identifications. The first urges a consideration of play as a sort of framing or tool that wrenches meaningful experience from an ongoing flow of action. It provides an untangling, a higher-order distancing, a reflective awareness. It draws its inspiration from a question that applies equally to all persons: What does it mean to be able to view the world from this high ground; what form of knowl-edge or structure of understanding is implicated or engendered from such height? On the other flank is pressure to understand play as an instrument of cultural connection, as a means of not only achieving a loftier point of view, but arriving there in the company of others. The question, in this instance, is specific to individuals who recognize and define one another by participating in common forms of communicative practice: What does it mean to view the world from this particular position, rather than some other one?

In attempting to provide at least provisional answers to these questions, I will argue that self and culture are both parts of a re-cursive process in which identities are "compendiously collected" and positioned in relation to others (Harré & van Langenhove, 1991). This is text construction and the process through which self and culture are mutually constituted and internally related. Interpo-lating, shared risks are read as play texts, as interpretive activity that constructs self and peer group identity. Borrowing from Harré, the result is the attainment of mindedness, or self-determination and re-flective awareness. This position is consistent with Vygotsky's (1971, 1979) argument that we develop into ourselves, and with Baldwin's (1906, 1911) statement that it is only through social life that we be-come relatively separate—relatively private and independent selves. It also finds expression in Geertz's (1986) reply to a question posed by Edward Young, an 18th-century aesthetician: "Born Originals," he asked, "how comes it to pass that we die Copies?" Geertz an-swered that it is the copying that orginates.

UNTANGLINGS AND ENTANGLEMENTS

The Mock Turtle of Alice's Wonderland described his lessons in Arithmetic as Ambition, Distraction, Uglification, and Derision, and provided an unexpected glimpse into the layers of meaning that children bind together as they construct their social environments. We can describe such layers in textual terms because they are created, maintained, and manipulated through semiotic means; because they define boundaries, rules, or constraints on acting; and because they can become decontextualized—lifted out of their communicative contexts to become objects of reflection in addition to instruments of communication (see Wertsch & Minick, 1990, for a similar discussion). In this regard, the decontexualizing quality of development—the increasing "freedom" from external control and social exigency—is perhaps better construed as a recontextualization on a higher plane of functioning.

The text is familiar territory for investigators of play, due largely to Bateson's (1972) insight that play is paradoxically text and context. Enclosed in "cheerful and irreverent quotation marks" (Bakhtin, 1981), the bite is but a nip; the blink is a wink. As with other modes of interpretive activity, play is at one and the same time "untanglings and entanglements" (Burke, 1966). The dialectical coordination of play and not-play provides a distance, transcendence, or second-level reflexivity. Thus, like language, art, and literature, play strives toward a more fully articulated and differentiated perspective through the refractive medium of expression.

Anthropologists and ethnographers have drawn most heavily upon the concept of "text" for understanding children's play, starting from the premise that play is a form of social commentary. Thus, they find gender stereotypes there (heroes and princesses), as well as social and family roles (doctors, mommies, and daddies). But beyond recreating social structures and institutions, children are considered to recreate themselves in play; not just anyone gets to play the daddy, and not everyone *has* to play the baby. It has been argued that children communicate about who they are in play, and that these self-descriptions also constitute acts of self-creation (e.g., Schwartzman, 1979).

Such ideas are fairly common in anthropological and ethnographic circles because these disciplines are sharply focused on persons as "culture-bearing" organisms. Anthropological approaches have been largely critical of traditional psychological research, arguing that it has placed too heavy an emphasis on children's play as a path to more mature and rational competencies. Drawing attention to "children's culture" as interesting in its own right and to be understood on its own terms, Huizinga (1938/1955) admonishes those who would approach play as a phenomenon transitional to more mature forms of functioning, as something that is not-yet-something-else. More recently, Sutton-Smith (1984) argues that a "natural science" approach to play (in contrast to an "interpretive science" approach) inappropriately intellectualizes and sanitizes the phenomenon, and reflects a Western cultural bias in which play, literature, and aesthetics have been subordinated to science, logic, and philosophy.

Perhaps such rationalist views have garnered empirical support because play is studied most often in highly supervised environments such as preschools, laboratories, and clinic playrooms. In these settings, teachers, therapists, and other adults purposively influence the direction of children's play. Themselves socialized into the cultural belief that play is children's work and handmaiden to developing social, linguistic, and cognitive competencies, the toys, games, and supervision adults provide channel children's behaviors toward "rational" objectives. But there are other types and contexts of play, which have been neglected by psychologists, that show it to be irrational, dysfunctional, mean spirited (Sutton-Smith, 1984), and a thing of power struggles, wounded feelings, and bloody noses. Some of the lessons learned in play are far removed from the social, language, and cognitive competencies studied by psychologists, although not unfamiliar, perhaps, to the lessons suffered by Lewis Carroll's Mock Turtle. These are good reasons, in any case, for re-examining conventional assumptions that the play realm is always rational, voluntary, spontaneous, and freely entered. Sutton-Smith (1984) argues the point most dexterously:

> [P]lay was often only free in the sense the players were free from the teacher to carry out their own particular kinds of terror. Most of the play on school playgrounds was made compulsory by one's peers. One substituted the authority of other children for the authority of adults. But then this is the way it has been throughout history where most village or tribal members have done what they had to in festival and game along with their fellows. Through the larger haul of

mankind's history such play has usually been obligatory. Defining it as voluntary is a twentieth-century ethnocentrism owing its origins to the contrast between leisure and factory work, and to the identification of the capacity to play with the privileges of elite groups. What distinguishes play from other frames of living is not any voluntariness, but rather its passionate and exciting character. Play is part of the Dionysian order of human expressiveness, rather than the Apollonian order of rationality. (pp. 75–76)

His excoriation takes careful and deliberate aim at the natural science or empirical–analytic paradigm, which holds that social science ought to model itself in theory and method after physical science. Much of the criticism is directed at a version of causality that maintains that antecedent causes can be distinguished from their consequent effects, that independent variables are distinct from dependent variables, and that having pinpointed such distinctions, behavior can be predicted and the universal laws that dictate behavior can be specified (Habermas, 1988; Harré & Madden, 1975; Koch, 1981; Lightfoot & Folds-Bennet, 1992; Secord, 1986; Valsiner, 1987).

Admittedly, the bulk of recent psychological play research is steeped in the mechanical cause–effect methodology that follows from the "natural science" approach. It focuses almost exclusively on the play of younger, especially preschool-age children, and its relationship to other developing social and cognitive competencies (see Rubin, Fein, & Vandenberg, 1983, for a thorough review). However, I am not prepared to join the roughshod ride over the past 100 years of developmental play research. As the interpretive paradigm gains influence in the discipline, so do perspectives espousing a view of play as interpretive activity. We shall find, in fact, a good deal of common ground between anthropological and developmental approaches. Although the latter have indeed been preoccupied with composing connections between play and rationality, it is not the objective and reductive *seeing-through* rationality suggested by the logico-empirical tradition, but a type of interpretive framing, a narrative knowing that Geertz (1986) describes as "*seeing-as* elucidations." It will be argued, finally, that play theory provides some clarity in regard to the developmental import and meanings of adolescents' risk involvement. First, however, a brief history of play, and efforts to undo it from the world of the serious.

A BRIEF HISTORY

Erikson (1963) understands play and rationality to form a beveled edge in the psychological development of the child. This is fore-shadowed in the title of his chapter "Toys and Reasons," which begins with an encounter between two boys whose activities illustrate the contrast between the worlds of work and leisure. The first is embodied in Tom Sawyer, who has been sentenced to whitewashing a fence on a fine spring day; the second in Ben Rogers, who is dramatizing a steamboat and all the mechanical parts and persons associated with its operation:

> He took up his brush and went tranquilly to work. Ben Rogers hove in sight presently—the very boy, of all boys, whose ridicule he had been dreading. Ben's gait was the hop-skip-jump—proof enough that his heart was light and his anticipations high. He was eating an apple, and giving a long, melodious whoop, at intervals, followed by a deep-toned ding-dong-dong, ding-dong-dong, for he was personating a steamboat. As he drew near, he slackened speed, took the middle of the street, leaned far over to starboard and rounded to ponderously and with laborious pomp and circumstance—for he was personating the *Big Missouri*, and considered himself to be drawing nine feet of water. He was boat and captain and engine-bells combined, so he had to imagine himself standing on his own hurricane-deck giving the orders and executing them:
> . . . "Stop the stabboard! Ting-a-ling-ling! Stop the labboard! Come ahead on the stabboard! Stop her! Let your outside turn over slow! Ting-a-ling-ling! Chow-ow-ow! Get out that head-line! *Lively* now! Come—out with your spring-line—what're you about there! Take a turn round that stump with the bight of it! Stand by that stage, now—let her go! Done with the engines, sir! Ting-a-ling-ling! *Sh't! sh't! sh't!*" (trying the gauge-cocks).
> Tom went on whitewashing—paid no attention to the steam-boat. Ben stared a moment, and then he said:
> "Hi-*yi*! *You're* a stump, ain't you! . . . You got to work, hey?" (cited in Erikson, 1963, pp. 209–210)

The contrasts between Tom's and Ben's activities are manifold. Tom works.[1] His behavior is dictated by a goal that extends beyond it and is imposed by another who occupies a position of authority over him. It is serious, purposive, rational, real. Ben's play, on the other hand, would seem to have no other goal than play itself. It is self-imposed, lacking in serious intent, fantastic, imaginative, and free. These contrastive components of work and play, or some subset of them, have provided psychologists with a base for theorizing about the functions of children's play, and the relationship between play and more serious-minded activities. Erikson used the episode above to make the point that play is an intermediate reality between fantasy and reality. As such, its purpose is to "hallucinate ego mastery and yet also to practice it." In playing the roles of captain and crew, gauge-cocks and engine, Ben creates a context of subjective control while simultaneously drawing upon the contents of the material world—its mechanical components as well as the people who construct and control them.

From this general psychoanalytic perspective, Erikson (1963) develops the thesis that play provides quiet harbor for egos that have been handled roughly. This understanding is fundamental to the enterprise of play therapy as it is used to diagnose and overcome real-world trauma. Those of us who have observed our children immunizing their dolls after a trip to the doctor's office, or sending them to their rooms for misbehaving, are hard pressed to deny that "reality," anxiously experienced, finds its way into the play arena. As a direct line from the personal and emotional to the rational world of real people and events, play seems to be a place for reflecting and repairing tattered egos. Its primary purpose is to create a context for mastering problems encountered outside of play, to transform passivity (being done to) into controlled activity.

Others have taken the position that rationality and play consti-

---

[1]Although the differences between Tom's and Ben's actions provide a convenient means for distinguishing between work and play, those very same differences point just as well to the slippage between them. Tom, after all, is only *pretending* to work. The coordination or interpenetration of work and play, fact and fantasy, taken-for-granted and speculative, is a recurring theme within the interpretive perspective.

tute entirely separate spheres of activity with differences so vast as to implicate different developmental functions. Greta Fein (1989), for example, argues that the child is of two minds, one literal and concerned with objective events and the logical relations that hold between them, the other nonliteral and concerned with emotionally charged subjective and mental events and their intuitive relations. By this reading, symbolic play is a product of the intuitive mind and serves affective rather than cognitive functions. In the same vein, others have suggested that children's linguistic forms and expressions not only vary in pretend versus nonpretend situations, but follow separate developmental trajectories (e.g., Garvey & Kramer, 1989).

The splitting off of play from other domains of functioning has interesting histories in science and culture. Our posture toward play, in fact, is every bit as ambivalent as it is toward adolescent risk-taking. The conflict concerns the nature of what is *enjoyable* for children versus what is *good* for them (Lightfoot & Valsiner, 1992; Wolfenstein, 1953). The Victorian age regarded play and art with a censorial eye. Guided by the moral code that "masturbation will make you mad," play was viewed as a form of autoeroticism whose deleterious effects were of comparable magnitude to the arousal that it induced. Moralists railed against thrills, excitations, and those "ticklings of sense" that were devoted to pleasure alone (Dewey, 1920/1957). Incidentally, during the late 19th century this attitude was dressed scientifically, and "excessive central nervous system excitation" became a matter of concern, not for moralists now, but for pediatricians and other child care experts. One odd consequence was the refurnishing of American nurseries with stationary cribs, rocking cradles having been expunged as instruments of excessive stimulation (see Valsiner, 1989).

This is just to foreshadow the point that Victorian attitudes did not pass without effect into the historical annals of a society that came to know better. In earlier times, the *good* and the *enjoyable* were antithetical. Sometime during the 1940s, however, the focus on children's autoeroticism was replaced with a concern for their need to explore the environment (Wolfenstein, 1953). Play became associated with motor development and exercise, and playgrounds were constructed to accommodate this newly discovered developmental "need" (Frost & Wortham, 1988; Lightfoot & Valsiner, 1992). With time, play was viewed not only as good for the child, but as an absolute necessity that ought to be part and parcel of mealtime, toilet training, school work, and all other domains of the child's activity *especially* if that activity could otherwise be construed as serious or unpleasant. Wolfenstein (1955) refers to the infusion of play into all other "serious" activities as the "fun morality." Thus, the serious should be made fun, and play should be taken seriously. But according to Wolfenstein, this "integration" is an elaborate deception, a modern redressing of puritanical defenses against impulses and the pleasure that comes from satisfying them:

> This defense would consist in diffusion, ceasing to keep gratification deep, intense, and isolated, but allowing it to permeate thinly through all activities. . . . Instead of the image of the baby who has fierce pleasures of autoeroticism and the dangerous titillation of rare moments of play, we get the infant who explores his world, every part of whose extent is interesting but none intensely exciting, and who may have a bit of harmless play thrown in with every phase of the day's routine. (Wolfenstein, 1955, p. 175)

It seems likely that these cultural conceptions contributed to the increased domestication of and adult involvement in, children's play. At the turn of the century parents and teachers began to supervise play and explicitly teach sports and games. The wide open fields surrounding school houses were marked off with fences and filled with gymnastic equipment—swings, bars, ladders, rings. Today practically all complex games played by children both in and out of school are organized by adults, and more than ever before, children's leisure time is spent in adult company. Even the "neighborhood group," the last group left free to develop a play life of its own, is threatened (in middle-class America, at least) by increasing mobility, dual income families, who meet the "child care problem" with a round of adult-supervised activities (sports teams, music lessons, extracurricular clubs), and care facilities. Time spent roaming the neighborhood with peers is diminishing, as is the suburban neighborhood itself. Even the architecture of modern homes reflects this change. Homes are no longer built for entertaining (witness the shrinking living and dining rooms), and most of the "living" takes place in the family room that often opens to an outdoor deck.

The house is thus oriented toward the back yard, usually fenced. In contrast, the suburban homes of the 1950s were generally described as focusing activity and attention toward the unfenced front yard, the primary location of children's group play (see Lemann, 1989).

FOLKLORE FORAY

Children's play and other cultural activities have become increasingly domesticated in this century, but the idea that adults can and should intrude in this domain for the purpose of imposing their own agenda is an ancient one that dates back at least to Plato's time. Plato argued that in order to establish a political system founded on rational principles of justice and ethical conduct, we must attend the myths, legends and tall tales of childhood, and bend them toward these higher aims:

> Shall we simply allow our children to listen to any stories that anyone happens to make up, and so to receive into their minds ideas often the very opposite of those we shall think they ought have when they are grown up? No, certainly not. It seems, then, our first business will be to supervise the making of fables and legends, rejecting all which are unsatisfactory; and we shall induce nurses and mothers to tell their children only those which we have approved, and to think more of molding their souls with these stories than they now do of rubbing their limbs to make them strong and healthy (cited in Cassirer, 1946, p. 72).

A professed enemy of myths, which he believed to embody irrationality and by extension the base and ignoble inclinations of human nature, Plato sought to purge political injustice by cleansing children's folklore. It may well be that children's souls are in some important sense molded by stories heard and told, but his belief in the intergenerational transmission of fables and legends is somewhat narrow and naive. Notwithstanding parental recitations of Mother Goose and Cinderella, "the scraps of lore which children learn from each other are at once more real, more immediately serviceable, and more vastly entertaining to them than anything which they learn from grown-ups" (Opie & Opie, 1959, p. 8). Indeed, much of the appeal of children's lore and play, much of its fun, lies in the fact that adults know nothing about it, or better, only suspect it, and disapprove. Indeed, this tendency toward separation and secrecy, the thrill of concealed intimacy—almost but not quite being caught—achieves its meridian in adolescent risk-taking.

In all of its manifestations, children's culture is marked by continuity and uniformity, yet remains nonetheless flexible to changing times and place. The Opies described it as a "continual process of wear and repair," because "like everything else in nature, [it] must adapt itself to new conditions if it is to survive" (1959, p. 9). And this culture's survival value (if we can call it that) is at least partially measured by how well it can stand as a declaration of identity, a provider of social cohesion, and an expression of feelings about important life events (e.g., Bronner, 1988; Sutton-Smith, 1981). Many of children's concerns endure across time and community, and this is apparent in long-whiskered stories, jokes, songs and rhymes that confront the prospects of sex, marriage, work, and, as below, sibling relations (collected by Herbert Golding, 1974; cited in Schwartzman, 1978, pp. 178–179):

> I had a little brother
> His name was Tiny Tim
> I put him in the washtub
> To teach him how to swim.
> He drank up all the water
> Ate up all the soap
> He died last night
> With a bubble in his throat.
>
> . . .
>
> Fudge, fudge call the judge
> Mamma's got a newborn baby
> Ain't no girl; ain't no boy
> Just a plain old baby
> Wrap it up in toilet paper
> Put it in the elevator
> First floor—miss
> second floor—miss
> Third floor—miss
> Fourth floor—kick it out the door.

Another well-played theme is student–teacher power relations. In much of it, power relations are reversed as teachers are bested by students, their authority challenged and caricatured. Surely no one is unfamiliar with this variation:

> Row, row, row your boat
> Gently down the stream
> Throw your teacher overboard
> And listen to her scream.

The following rhyme trashes arithmetic as well as the teacher:

> Four and four are twenty-four
> Kick the teacher out the door
> If she squeals, bring her in,
> Hang her on a safety pin.
> (reported in Sutton-Smith, 1981, p. 256)

Jokes, too, parody classroom lessons and pedagogy:

There was this class and the teacher was asking the kids questions. She asked one little boy, "What's round and red and grows on a tree and has green leaves?" Little Johnny says, "The pear." The teacher says, "No, Johnny, it's an apple." But since he said it was round and it does grow on a tree, she said, "That just goes to show you that you're thinking right." She goes on and asks a few more students the same question. Well about that time Peter, who was a smart-ass, sitting in the back of the room, yells out, "Teacher, I've got one for you. What do I have in my pocket that I've got my hand ahold of that's long, white, and thin, and has a red head?" And the teacher says, "Oh Peter!" And he says, "No teacher, it's not, it's a matchstick, but that just goes to show you you're thinking right." (reported in Bronner, 1988, p. 133)

Clearly there is no dearth of material to illustrate that children reveal what matters to them in story, play, humor, and rhyme, and all of it speaks to the fundamental refulgence of folklore. The forms and objects of children's play, their jokes and rhymes, stories and slang are elucidations of their lives. This would seem to be the primary purpose: elucidation—the clarity of perspective that obtains in the course of putting one's experience into circulation, in constructing a text (see also Lightfoot, in press-a). As argued previously, all interpretive activity strains in this direction.

PLAY'S PARADOX

Gregory Bateson's (1972) theory of metacommunication constitutes a prototype for contemporary efforts to carve a position for play in the edifice of interpretive theory. Inspired by the apparent meta-communication (i.e., messages about how other messages should be interpreted—"this nip is not a bite; this is play") that he observed in young monkeys, Bateson formulated a theory in which the ability to play betokens an evolutionary mutation in the ability to communicate, in particular, the discovery of map–territory relations. His argument is that the relationship between language and the objects it denotes is comparable to that between a map and its territory. They are of different logical types—the word "cat" cannot scratch us (p. 180). But the paradox of play, made much of in the psychological and anthropological literature, lies in the interdependence of map and territory: "[P]lay implies a special combination of primary and secondary processes. . . . In primary process, map and territory are equated; in secondary process, they can be discriminated. In play, they are both equated and discriminated" (p. 185).

Bateson argued that through play, children learn that behavior can be framed, logically typed and styled. By this reading, what is instrumental to development is not so much the learning of the particular style or role—mommy, daddy, doctor, dragon—but rather, the learning of "stylistic flexibility and the fact that the choice of style or role is related to the frame and context of behavior" (1972; p. 149). It is not the case, in other words, that children simply pour themselves into and out of and thereby learn the shape of these social forms and idioms. From Bateson's position, play shows its value as a carefully scripted conflation of logical types. Nevertheless, where his theoretic agenda was explicitly epistemological, much of the anthropological literature that has followed in his wake is intended to reveal the intermingling of sociocultural forms and children's personal experience; that is, it turns its hand toward issues of cultural identification (e.g., Schwartzman, 1978).

In many of these sorts of studies, children are observed to represent particular social roles in their play. Moreover, the orchestration of it all, who plays which role, and who decides, is seen as substantially constrained by the children's interpersonal histories with one another. Helen Schwartzman (1978) noted, for example, that

> [t]he roles that children adopt, or are assigned, frequently reflect the authority structure of the play group (e.g., the mother dominates the baby and defines activities for him/her to engage in—e.g., "Now it's time for you to go to sleep"), and at the center, they often reflected the hierarchy of children outside the play sphere (e.g., those who frequently played "mothers" and "fathers" were often the most popular and desired "friends" in the classroom). In house play, the role of the pet (e.g., "kitty," "doggie") was generally assumed by one of the more unpopular children in the group. (p. 239)

Similar conditions prevail in the play of African children: Only older boys take the role of the chief; only the most unpopular play the role of the village villain (Centner, 1962; cited in Schwartzman, 1978).

The manner by which extant interpersonal relationships become manifest in play is also apparent in the jokes and humor used by Western adolescents in their peer interactions. Sanford and Eder (1984) found that forms of humor varied according to the interpersonal contexts of use. Memorized jokes occur frequently between acquaintances (rather than close friends), and in mixed-sex and mixed-age groups. They display a "sophisticated" identity through prohibited expressions and knowledge of sexuality, intercourse, genitalia, and menstruation. Joke-tellers gain the attention and admiration of others. Funny stories, on the other hand, are shared primarily between close friends. Usually the narrator or a close friend is featured as a central character engaged in some rule-violating activity. Practical jokes, a third form of adolescent humor, comment on social relationships in a more personal manner. Because they can show either friendship or dislike for particular individuals, they are often ambiguous and framing them as "play" can be a complicated affair:

> Lisa then played a trick on Wendy. She tiptoes all the way around the table and then she stood behind Wendy and put her index finger to her mouth, telling everyone to be quiet and not let Wendy know that

she was behind her. And she didn't [know] . . . because another girl was standing next to her talking to her. And then Lisa dropped a piece of wrapper into Wendy's milk, which made Wendy turn real red and made her more angry than anything else. Wendy first turned to Renee and said, "Do you have 20 cents I could borrow to buy a new milk?" And finally Wendy turned to Lisa and said, "Lisa, give me 20 cents to buy a new milk." And then Lisa said, "Here, you can have my milk." And at that point Wendy laughed a little bit about it. (p. 240)

The labile though nonetheless tightly woven relationship between map and territory is illuminated further by Grahame and Jardine's (1990) analysis of adolescents' "mucking about" in the classroom. They begin with a critique of Willis's seminal study of working-class boys (*Learning to Labour*, 1977). Extending the Marxian notion of class struggle to the naughty behavior of teenagers, Willis argued that "having a laff" in class is a conscious confrontation with middle-class values that dramatizes working-class subculture. Classroom disruptions are thus conceived as a form of resistance against a society that simultaneously insists on the middle-class dream (e.g., owning a home or business, pursuing higher education) but fails to provide the resources necessary for achieving it (see also Baron's [1989] study of the street culture of punks). However, Grahame and Jardine took issue with the clash-of-separate-cultures perspective as being overly utilitarian. To focus too narrowly on class struggle is to overlook the ludic character of such behavior (see also Corrigan, 1979). They offered the synthetic concept of "playful resistance" as an alternative.

The concept was illustrated in analyses of communicative interchanges that took place within a ninth-grade boys' home economics class (Grahame & Jardine, 1990). The semester was devoted to textiles, and included a session on "tufted fabrics." Needless to say, this subject proved to be fertile ground for exploring the interstices of the teacher's lesson and a shadow lesson constructed by the students. The official agenda was to draw the class into a discussion about the uses of tufted fabrics. The students held up their end of the lesson and responsibly answered the teacher's questions and prompts by providing many examples of tufted things, including jackets, glove linings, and fuzzy slippers. Over the course of the session, however, they developed a separate, although playfully connected stream of discourse that included see-through nightgowns, edible underwear, whips, muzzles, and a discussion of the number of beavers it takes to make a jacket. Importantly, the official and unofficial "lessons" were characterized as flowing into each other rather than being independent and disconnected. "[T]here are two contexts for responses," wrote Grahame and Jardine (1990), and children occupy them simultaneously, use them in fact, to create a special unity—play:

> We think there may be some point in viewing this production as a kind of resistance, but it is a resistance of a peculiar sort. It corresponds neither to the systematic inversion of school values, nor to the willful disruption of educational communication described by subcultural theorists. Nor does it involve a well-defined withdrawal into territories outside of school control. Instead, the aside is so closely articulated to the lesson structure that students must keep in constant touch with the main movement of the lesson to achieve their artful digressions. In a peculiar way, the aside depends on fine attunement to the official structure of the lesson. . . . Inasmuch as the aside production involves collaboration to create enjoyable interludes that neither ignore nor arrest the lesson's progress, we are inclined to see it as a species of playful resistance. What is being resisted is not so much knowledge of fabrics per se, but rather the requirement to take fully seriously the collective attention being given to that knowledge in a classroom context. What is being affirmed is the pleasure of skillful probing of lesson topics for their comic potential, and this probing remains, in an important sense, "on topic." (pp. 299–300)

Grahame and Jardine's depiction of the player as one who assumes a double role reminds us again of the duality of play and the way that it forms and clarifies what lies beneath the surface—peer relations (friendly or not), social roles and stereotypes, teacher–student relations, the historical record in general. The player, however, does not act in consignment to this record. Play is no hollow echo of past experience, no casual acquiescence to habit and expectation. Contrariwise, it regards experience, habit, expectation from a higher ground and from there presents the key to its own meaning.

The work presented here also indicates, importantly, that not all meanings are equally transparent or deep. Lisa's practical joke, opaque and awkward, stands in counterpoint to the artful digressions of the home economics students. The vast variety of play types and joke types testifies to the importance of sharing play's high ground, and how the ability to do so is socially and historically constrained. Memorized jokes, for example, are common among mixed-sex acquaintances, whereas funny personal stories dominate the humor of close friends. Both forms involve a self-display, but in the first case it is oblique, and "sophisticated" knowledge about sexuality and so forth is expressed through "stories" of fictional characters. In the latter case, however, the central characters are personal—self or friends—and communicate knowledge of and allegiance to peer and adult norms. Memorized jokes, moreover, have frames more easily read and recognized (e.g., "Didja hear the one about . . . ?") than those belonging to personal stories and especially practical jokes, which undoubtedly contributes to their popularity among individuals who don't know each other well. In other words, although play is always personally and interpersonally illuminating, it varies in the extent to which this is so. It may light just the surface of things and show an ongoing shifting of mood, intention, and understanding, or it may show the deeper desires and definitions of self.

DEEP PLAY

Geertz (1972) elaborates such an issue in applying the concept of "deep play" to the Balinese cockfight. By their own accounts, the men of Bali are "cock crazy." Geertz describes their cockfights as a "popular obsession of consuming power." His analysis focuses on how gambling is used as a device for creating interesting, or "deep" matches. The depth of the match depends on the size of the center bet. Large-bet fights include the finest quality animals, and great care is taken to ensure that they are evenly matched so as to maximize unpredictable outcomes. If one is agreed to be of better size or condition, or more pugnacious than his competitor, his spurs may be positioned at a less advantageous angle by an individual well trained in such handicapping. Deep play, then, is that in which the stakes are so high, and the outcome so unpredictable, that it makes no sense to participate at all. That is, in the case of a fortune waged on an even bet, the marginal utility of what could be won is much less than the marginal disutility of what stands to be lost. Bentham (1802/1931) coined the term "deep play" in the 17th century, and argued that it is immoral and should be legally sanctioned because only the irrational—addicts, fools, and children—play these games, and they should be protected from themselves. Geertz argues, however, that a utilitarian perspective misses the essential point. The depth of play is not indexed by cost–benefit ratios, but by the extent to which play references social realities that extend beyond it. His analysis shows that the "deepest" fights, those involving the most money and the least predictability, are those that most closely simulate the social matrix and power structure of Balinese life. Under such conditions, the cockfight reaches most deeply into the contexts of everyday life, and it is from here that it derives its consuming power and aesthetic sense. It is an expressive form, essentially, that interprets and objectifies a particular social reality. As Geertz notes, it is "only apparently cocks that are fighting there. Actually it is men."

Much of the interview material presented in the next chapter suggests that adolescents' risk involvement falls into the category of deep play (see also Sutton-Smith & Kelly-Byrne, 1984). The teenagers indicated, first of all, that much of the appeal of risk-taking lies in the uncertainty of the outcome, usually (but not always) expressed in terms of "getting caught." In the words of a 17-year-old, the thrill, the "rush," lies in "almost but not quite getting caught." What is most interesting, however, is not that the teenagers self-consciously pursue these sorts of experiences, but that they tend to organize them so that they may be shared. Although it was universally acknowledged that friends are impressed by those who attempt the extraordinary, risks were not construed as a simple attention-getting device, but as social commentaries that express and transform interpersonal relationships. They demonstrate "your commitment to the group"; they "show what lengths you'll go to to be with your friends"; they "bring you closer because you've survived an ordeal together," "because you have a secret that you share." Discussions of their own risk involvement were replete with examples of how high adventure, socially shared, is demonstrative of interpersonal relationships and desires: "[Getting drunk] is a good excuse to fall over that cute guy you really like"; "[skipping school] makes you closer because you feel like you've survived an ordeal together—you've beat the establishment together"; "[stealing a case of beer from a delivery truck] shows what lengths you'll go to to be with the group"; "[taking LSD] is a different way to relate, a different way of being close." In the eyes of the teenagers interviewed, play is most meaningful and acquires its depth not because of risk per se, but because of what is communicated to others by proceeding in spite of it. Thus, the ability to play, and especially to play deeply, has much to do with understanding, expressing, and developing one's self in relation to others.

We have come considerable distance toward understanding the expressive potential of play, but its generative power remains a dim outline. This task falls to developmental psychologists, rightly and squarely, if not always comfortably. The following pages present an overview of a rather small family of developmental theories. All of them share the axiomatic foundations of the organismic paradigm, and all are plumbed for their capacity to illuminate the constructive, semiotic, and temporally organized aspects of play. Informed by modern interpretive insights, these theories extend an invitation to consider adolescent risk-taking as a form of play that unites personal meanings and peer cultural forms, and contributes to the development and constitution of both.

DEVELOPMENTAL PERSPECTIVES

Piaget's Project

In his widely cited volume *Play, Dreams and Imitation in Childhood*, Piaget (1962) undertakes an extensive project to bring play within the purview of his general theory of cognitive development. In contrast to much of his later work, the play project reveals a psychoanalytic influence in which play is understood to protect the ego from "forced accommodations" in everyday life (see also Nicolopolou, 1993). From this perspective, children produce in their play conditions for mastering what is ordinarily denied them by virtue of more powerful others. However, Piaget's interpretation of play is importantly different from Freud's (and most other play theorists' for that matter) because he believes that the mastery attending it is illusory. Play has no bearing on reality, moves away from it, in fact, thus making no contribution whatsoever to further intellectual developments. This is not to say that the material world is absent from the play arena: "We can be sure that all the happenings, pleasant or unpleasant, in the child's life will have repercussions on her dolls," but "the doll only serves as an opportunity for the child to re-live symbolically her own life in order to assimilate more easily its various aspects as well as to resolve daily conflicts and realise unsatisfied desires" (p. 107).

Within Piaget's general equilibration theory, organism–environment interactions that equally engage assimilation and accommodation processes constitute the hallmark of mature and fully adaptive thought. In the young organism, however, they are rarely coordinated so elegantly. At times accommodation predominates and imitation comes to the fore; at other times assimilation has the upper hand and the child plays. It would thus appear that from a bird's eye view of ontogeny, Piaget had it in mind eventually to synthesize play and imitation to the more mature functioning of adaptive thought; "In so far as intelligence, imitation and play are considered . . . , imitation is a continuation of accommodation, play a continuation of assimilation, and intelligence a harmonious combination of the two" (1962, p. 104). Oddly, despite his apparent allegiance to a necessary synthesis, he was clear and emphatic that play constitutes a domain unto itself—a singular domain for a solitary player—that has no bearing on later emerging developments. The function of assimilation is simply to preserve and consolidate existing competencies.

It is obvious here that the mind is most unyielding to the effects of the material world during bouts of play: "Unlike objective thought, which seeks to adapt itself to the requirements of external reality, imaginative play is a symbolic transposition which subjects things to the child's activity, without rules or limitation. It is therefore almost pure assimilation, i.e., thought polarised by preoccupation with individual satisfaction" (1962, p. 87). The lawless, hedonistic, and highly circumscribed world of play is particularly apparent in Piaget's discussion of group play. He would undoubtedly disapprove of the term "group play," would consider it a misnomer to the extent that it implies any negotiation or coconstruction of a shared play reality. Even in the company of others, the play world remains idiosyncratic—socially impotent and impregnable. Impotent because the child is aware that ludic symbols have been created for personal purposes, that they are symbols for the self, not others, and there is consequently no serious effort to enforce them on others; impregnable because the entry of others into the child's symbolic universe either reinforces a belief in the subjective illusion, or destroys it entirely. This is seen in the culmination of play's development, games with rules. These are social realities that have been negotiated between "equals and contemporaries" whose shared participation implies an ability and willingness to subordinate ego to reality. In becoming collective, play looses its imaginative content, that is, its symbolism, and is supplanted by adaptive intelligence (1962, p. 144).

Contemporary investigators of play have raised several objections to Piaget's conclusions. One concerns the idea that play is diminished as thought becomes more realistic and adaptive (e.g., Bretherton, 1989; Sutton-Smith, 1966). Bretherton, for example, made the point that children's play becomes more fantastic, rather than realistic, as they mature: "With a firmer grip on reality," she argued, children "find a variety of guises under which to enact emotionally significant themes of caring and aggression, of authority and obedience, of danger and power, of pain, of growth and change, of puzzlement and of fun" (pp. 395–396). We also have good reason to cast a doubtful eye on his depiction of play groups as collectives of "equals." It is now recognized widely that play groups are not composed of equals, and that the asymmetries of social relationships are often instantiated in play interactions. Play does not seem to be the wild romp of subjectivity that Piaget suggested, or a wanton "assimilation of reality to the ego." There is much about it that is neither capricious nor without rules or limitations.

Most significant, however, is that Piaget's version of play as essentially undaunted by the material world and unchecked by accommodative processes strips it of any possible role in the child's development. A number of psychologists who, unlike Piaget, consider play as a source of novelty and variation (e.g., Buck-Morss, 1987; Vygotsky, 1977; Winnicott, 1971) argue that structures of action organized in play come into conflict with the organization of nonplay experiences. In playing, children confront the difference between objects and their symbolic representations (e.g., riding a pony or a broomstick); they confront the difference between behavior and the roles that organize or dictate behavior (e.g., being a sister or pretending to be a sister). Children's language games (Topsy-Turvies, puns, riddles) are thought to reflect and contribute to an awareness of the difference between language use and rules of language use (Buck-Morss, 1987). All of these examples illustrate how children create contexts in which they distance themselves from the matrix of nonplay experience, and temporarily suspend perceived rules and roles, limits and constraints that structure and give meaning to actions and objects. The developmental implications are that in bringing to imaginative realization what is normally obscured from view (to paraphrase Geertz, 1927), children gain control of the organization of their own behavior. That is, they become conscious of rules and roles, and with this comes the potential for active manipulation and intentional transformation. Within Piaget's (1962) theory, however, such awareness only occurs in the presence of accommodation: "While accommodation of thought is generally conscious, because external or internal obstacles call forth consciousness, assimilation, even when rational, is usually unconscious" (p. 172).

On the other hand, there is much about Piaget's theory of play and imitation that has received little attention from his detractors, but deserves further scrutiny because it contains his most coherent statement of the link between play and imitation. Although the eventual synthesis he envisioned with the advent of fully adapted thought was poorly effected in his presentation, we can hound some measure of sensibility from his discussion of their common heritage—the image.

Piaget launches into an extended discussion of the image in the course of describing the early differentiation of play and imitation. The image is the interior copy or reproduction of the object, an "interior symbol." Piaget argues emphatically that the image is not an exact replica of the object imitated; it is not a "mere continuation of perception," but a "construction akin to that which produces the schemas of intelligence." Although the image takes its material from the world of sensation, the act of imitating changes the imaged object fundamentally. Thus, the material is not only sensorial (from the world of sensation), but motor (from the act of imitating): "The ability to reproduce a tune which has been heard makes the inner hearing of it infinitely more precise, and the visual image remains vague if it cannot be drawn or mimed. The image is as it were the draft of potential imitation" (1962, p. 70).

When Piaget speaks of the image as a potential draft for future imitations, he has it in mind to describe a tendency toward a clarifying exteriorization. Images, or interior symbols, vary in their tendencies to be exteriorized. Some involve a "larger part of true interiorization" (i.e., tend less toward exteriorization) and remain individual because they constitute a translation of personal experiences. This includes the ludic symbol and, in the most extreme form, the unconscious symbol. The other end of the symbolic continuum is anchored by more fully collectivized symbols and signs. Interior speech, for example, which is both the interiorization of acquired exterior speech as well as the draft of words to come, always retains a tendency toward exteriorization because it is more socialized than other symbol types. In this latter case, the image may

> constitute a draft for new exteriorizations. It may again display itself in imitations, both of people and things, in drawing and plastic techniques, in rhythms and sounds, dances and rituals, in language itself, where, in the form of the "affective language" discovered and analyzed by Bally, the power of expression is enhanced by resorting to the image and the symbol. But in order to understand the future destinies of the image and of symbolic representation, which as we have seen are provided by imitation with the wherewithal to make more or less accurate copies of reality, it will be necessary to study the counterpart of imitation, i.e., play and imaginative construction, which will make use of these copies in very varying ways, endowing them with meanings ever more remote from their imitative point of departure. (1962, p. 72)

The rest of his story—about how play is invested with personal meanings and idiosyncratic symbols, about its hedonistic reverie and ultimate usurpation by collective and rule-governed games—has already been told. But it was a poor denouement for such a brilliant first act. The consequence of harnessing play to assimilation, imitation to accommodation, and adapted, objective thought to their coordination, was to impose a categorical distinction that was theoretically incoherent. However, his discussion of the general interior symbol (rather than the ludic symbol in particular) as a potential draft of future exteriorizations provides some leeway for considering play as interpretive activity. By this reading, the personal meanings expressed in play are made intelligible as they take collective form. As the drafts of things to come, they constitute preadaptations, preunderstandings, or tendencies that are developed and articulated in the course of creating the play text. Thus, instead of being an unsophisticated, distorting precursor to objective thought, play is a mode of activity that complements it. In certain ways similar to the objectivity gained by mature and balanced reasoning, play strives to step out of the realm of immediate and unreflective action, and put it all into perspective. It becomes a "strategy for encompassing situations" (Burke, 1966), or for defining "situations of involvement" (Taylor, 1985).

Because play, from this perspective, is constrained by objects, influences, and meanings that exist outside the magical control of subjectivity, it takes on consequences for development. Whereas Piaget was able to argue that because play is free, the mastery attending it must be illusory, the alternative presented here has it that the mastery is real because the freedom is illusory. This is particularly apparent in theories that consider play as a unique relationship between what is subjective and what is socially shared.

Transitional Phenomena

Winnicott (1971) writes of a transitional space between inner/subjective and outer/objective realities in which play, and later cultural experience, are uniquely located. He posits a developmental progression that begins with the infant's "transitional object"—its first symbol and psychological possession—its attachment to, for example, a teddy bear, a doll, or a piece of cloth. This first possession (and he insists that it is a *possession*, not an object per se) is transitional in a double sense. First, it defines an "intermediate area" between personal psychic reality and objective shared reality. Second, it provides a means of negotiating between the two, of separating the subjective me from the objective not-me. In this sense, it is transitional between "object-relating," in which case the object is a "bundle of projections" under magical control, and the use and control of actual objects that belong to an external and shared reality. The transitional object symbolizes a union between the two, a pivot around which to define the boundaries of self and not-self.

Extending his idea of transition objects to transitional phenomena in general, Winnicott argues that they chart a journey from the purely subjective to objectivity, a "journey of progress toward experiencing": "We experience life in the area of transitional phenomena, in the exciting interweave of subjectivity and objective observation, and in an area that is intermediate between the inner reality of the individual and the shared reality of the world that is external to individuals" (p. 64).

Clearly, transitional phenomena were considered relevant beyond infancy and the early emerging capacity to distinguish between self and other. Winnicott (1971) writes that "[t]here is a direct development from transitional phenomena to playing and from playing to shared playing, and from this to cultural experiences" (p. 51). In all cases, the individual gathers objects from external reality in the service of inner, personal reality, and in so doing invests them with personal meanings. But Winnicott emphasizes repeatedly that subjective and objective phenomena are bound to one and the same dialectical process. Personal meanings do not "cause" objective reality: "[P]rojective mechanisms assist in the act of *noticing what is there*, but they are not the *reason why the object is there*" (p. 90; original italics). Projection, then, is not hallucinatory, but fosters attentiveness to the material world—the object was there, waiting to be constructed. This is, according to Winnicott, the paradox of transitional phenomena: "the baby creates the object, but the object was there waiting to be created and to become a cathected object" (p. 89). Recursively connected, each explains the other and forms an essential and irreducible part of an interpretive whole.

Baldwin pursues a like-minded analysis with similar results. His theory of play is located within a broader theory of genetic logic (Baldwin, 1906), and eventually forms the basis of an explication regarding the relationship between aesthetics and knowledge (Baldwin, 1911). In the first volume of *Thought and Things* (1906), he describes play as conscious self-illusion, or a conscious "oscillation between inner and outer." The play situation reinstates the common meanings of "outer" social organization, but the player is aware that the construction is imaginative, that play "stands for" reality. Thus, "consciousness, even while busy with the play objects, casts sly glances behind the scenes, making sure that its firm footing of reality is not entirely lost."

The oscillation between inner and outer is construed by Baldwin as a merging of two essentially opposed methods of control: The inner control of personal meaning contributes to a sense of agency, personal detachment, and what Baldwin called a "don't have to" attitude. But although it is selective in this regard, it always takes place against a backdrop of socially agreed upon (and imposed) "facts." Play thus has the character of being fact as well as meaning, and it is this duality, the union of the "semblant" and the factual, that fosters development on both fronts. The unifying process is that of "feeling into" the play object, and is comparable to Lipps's (1903) *einfuhlung* (translated to *empathy* by Titchener in 1910), which describes projections of affect onto artistic symbols. In case of both play and art, the process entails "making an object, for present and personal purposes, *what it might be*; and being for 'personal purposes,' it takes on, in a great variety of cases, personal form" (Baldwin, 1906, p. 124). The essence of play, Baldwin continues, is that it is simultaneously *experimental* and *selective*:

> The play object does not mean an individual in the same sense that a memory object proper does. It is an "experimental" object. It is held and controlled with the express psychic proviso or reservation that its meaning is yet to be made up. It is constructed, but not assigned; it subsists, but does not yet have a sphere of existence. The individuation, therefore, just at the time of the play function, is one that reads what may be called "experimental meaning" into an image: holds it as an object fit for, and so far standing for, *alternative meanings*. It is this construction, essentially characteristic of the play-mode, and of the higher semblant or art consciousness, that I propose to call the *Schema*. (p. 165; original italics)

Because the play situation is a personal selection (involving the "don't have to" attitude), Baldwin considered it fundamental to the development of self—the development of control and inner determination in particular: Play is the pursuit of *"an interest which isolates the context from its external setting and distinctly negatives [sic] its external control.* The semblant context thus satisfies a germinating interst in a detached and self-controlled meaning" (p. 120; original italics). This is perhaps most apparent in Baldwin's description of "playing at being a self":

> The striking impulse to "show-off," the "self-exhibiting" impulse—made much of, and quite properly so, in the literature of both play

and art—also carries on the sembling motive. This impulse is, of course, directly socializing; and when indulged consciously, it is directly social. But it also means the setting up of a show-person, motivated not by actual normal function, but by artificial and experimental make-believe, in the presence of another who is the spectator at the exhibition. Moreover, its content is always imitative of actual self-material (hence the term *inner imitation*). It is a show-self, made up for the purpose. (1906, p. 125)

In play, then, we observe tentative and prospective reconstructions of self, an exteriorization of hypothetical and experimental meanings that are nevertheless closely articulated to the "actual," the "real," the taken-for-granted.

The developmental import of play as a controlled or controlling situation is the vertex of Vygotsky's analysis. He writes that "a child's greatest self-control occurs in play" (1977, p. 92), because, in play, action is subordinated to meaning—to the rules and constraints of an imaginary situation. "In play the child is free," he says, "but this is an illusory freedom," subject to the imaginary situation, or the rules of the game, and this is where play becomes developmentally significant. In particular, Vygotsky (1977) argues that in play, children organize a zone of proximal development:

> The play–development relationship can be compared with the instruction–development relationship, but play provides a background for changes in needs and in consciousness of a much wider nature. Play is the source of development and creates the zone of proximal development. Action in the imaginative sphere, in an imaginary situation, the creation of voluntary intentions and the formation of real-life plans and volitional motives—all appear in play. (p. 96)

This statement encapsulates Vygotsky's main thesis regarding play as development's leading edge. The essence of play is its transitional nature between situationally constrained behavior and "thought that is totally free of real situations" (i.e., general, abstract knowledge). Wrenching meaning from situations is not yet possible for the young child and requires a "pivot." For example, in order to imagine a horse at all, the child needs to imagine a horse contained in a stick. The stick, the material pivot, fixes meaning, and prevents it from evaporating. But the pivot cannot be a neutral object. Whereas adults can let anything "stand for" a horse, this is not the

case for children, although Vygotsky claimed that it becomes so because of their play. We have then, Vygotsky's version of play's paradox, "a highly interesting contradiction . . . in which the child operates with meanings severed from objects and actions (e.g., horses
and sticks), but in real action with real objects operates with them in
fusion" (p. 89). This marks play as transitional from operating with
an alienated meaning in a real situation to operating with meanings
free of real situations.

The illusory freedom of the imaginary situation implicates a
second paradox that Vygotksy relates more fully to the development
of motives and desires. Because play presumes a willing submission
to the rules of the situation, it defines a path of greatest and least resistance. It is in an important sense self-determined, or what Baldwin would call self-selective, but also creates demands to act against
impulse. As such, "play gives the child a new form of desires, i.e.,
teaches him to desire by relating his desires to a fictitious 'I'—to his
role in the game and its rules" (1977, p. 92). So in subjecting one's
self to the rules of the game, one comes to desire them. The rule becomes an affect.

Dorothy Holland (1991) has recently applied Vygotsky's theory
of play to explain how romantic relationships are socially constructed by undergraduate women. The question she addressed is a central one for cultural anthropology (her own discipline), but also for
social science in general: How do cultural systems direct and moti-
vate people's actions? She extended Vygotsky's notion of a rule-governed imaginary situation to cultural models of romance, and argued that in the process of acting within the romantic sphere,
cultural systems become internalized and organize thoughts and
emotions. Her longitudinal study of women's developing expertise
and involvement in romantic relationships provides compelling evidence for the claim that the meanings of cultural systems, and the
desire to participate in them, are developmentally conjoined and
emerge in cultural activity.

THE CASE OF ADOLESCENCE

At end of his chapter on play, Vygotsky makes the comment that
play is most significant during the preschool years. At other ages, it

is "serious" either because the imaginary situation is not separated from the real one, as is the case for very young children, or because it is "converted into internal processes" of inner speech and abstract thought, in the case of older children. An example of this conversion is provided in an earlier paper on adolescent play (1931), recently translated and published by van der Veer and Valsiner (1994). In an argument strikingly similar to Winnicott's, adolescent imagination and fantasy are presented as a link in a continuous chain extending from the play of young children, to the creative literary and scientific work of adults. Vygotsky extends the play theories of Wundt and Spranger to suggest that adolescent imagination is play without action. It reveals, clarifies, gives direction and control:

> When the poet says: "I will dissolve in tears over this fiction," he realizes that this figment is something unreal, but his tears belong to the realm of reality. In this way an adolescent finds a means of expressing his rich inner emotional life and his impulses in fantasy. But it is also in fantasy that he is able to discover an effective means of finding a direction for this emotional life and for taking charge of it. Similar to the way in which an adult overcomes his feelings during the reading of a literary work, say of a lyric poem, the adolescent clarifies, reveals to himself and incorporates his emotions and his longings in creative images. The unexpressed part of his life finds its expression in creative images. (Vygotsky, 1994, p. 284)

Vygotsky's paper on adolescent fantasy not only predates his explication of preschoolers' play, but contains the kernel of what he would later develop as his theory of the zone of proximal development—the intersection of objective, social relations, and subjective, personal relations that forms the bedrock of future actions and developments:

> Objective expression may be coloured by vivid emotional tones, but subjective fantasies are also often observed within the sphere of objective creativity. To illustrate the rapprochement of both of these channels in the development of the imagination, we should like to point out that it is, precisely, within the realm of his fantasy that, for the first time, the adolescent has a chance to discover the course his life is to take. His strivings and obscure drives are cast in the mould of specific images. In his fantasy, he anticipates his future and conse-

quently also comes closer to its creative construction and realization. (Vygotsky, 1994, p. 285)

Bringing Vygotsky's theory of play into the light of modern interpretive perspectives reveals a twofold focus on epistemological matters as well as issues of sociocultural identifications, that is, an explication of play as both untanglings and entanglements. The idea that play is a means of achieving a higher-order perspective, a way of stepping out of one's predicament, is readily apparent in his notion of illusory freedom; "what passes unnoticed by the child in real life becomes a rule of behavior in play." Vygotsky's greatest contribution to our understanding, however, lies in his suggestion that these epistemic issues are related to sociocultural concerns: The self-restraint, self-determination, and reflective awareness engendered by play create a new form of desires, new motives for acting, which are harnessed to the fictive self and which "tomorrow will become her basic level of real action and morality."

What may now be said of adolescent risk-taking and peer culture? During adolescence, the games, stories, humor, and rhyme of childhood lose their power to communicate and clarify the sense of who one is or would like to be. The teenager constructs new signs of the self, fashions new amulets to which cleave peer culture and social identity. Modes of dress, professed ideals, music choices, drug preferences, and other risk activities: These are the transitional objects of adolescence. They are imaginative constructions, moulds into which they cast desire, markers of that potent place in which action becomes meaningful as cultural experience. The next two chapters are presented as an empirical demonstration of this general point of view. In particular, and from an interpretive perspective, adolescents' social dramas and adventures are read as play texts, which are constructed, semiotically mediated, and temporally organized. They will be explored as a medium through which self and peer group identities are constituted, as texts in which to inscribe desires and affections, and position oneself at the threshold of a story.

CHAPTER 5

Adolescent Risk-Taking as Transformative Experience

INTERVIEWER: What's appealing about taking risks?

17-YEAR-OLD: That's how you grow up—experiences. The only way to get experience is to take risks. When you're growing up you've got to find out—"Well, I've heard all this stuff about sex and drugs and driving"—and you have to try out a little bit of everything and from that build your own plan, your own lifestyle, and become the person you are when you become developed.

16-YEAR-OLD: I think growth—inner growth. And a feeling of independence and maturity in trying something new. Even if I fail, I still kind of pat myself on the back and say, "Hey, you tried it, and no one can blame you for sitting back and not participating." I want to be a participant.

These two teenagers are perhaps more eloquent than most, but their faith in some connection between risk-taking and their own development is fairly typical. In the first case, risks provide a special type of experience instrumental to personal growth; they are building blocks for the construction of self. This is implicit in the second response as well, in which risks are associated with inner growth, and feelings of independence and maturity. But whereas the first teenager is inclined toward a view of risks as particular, bounded events that somehow coalesce into a lifestyle, the second emphasizes the importance of effort. Simply *trying* something new has its own rewards; regardless of outcome, it convinces him of his own active participation, agency, and self-conscious desire to "move something along toward an open future" (Erikson, 1965, p. 11).

The material presented in this chapter has been extracted from a variety of sources, including responses to a paper-and-pencil checklist, speculations regarding the risk-taking of hypothetical story characters, answers to general questions about what constitutes and motivates risk-taking, as well as stories about personal risk involvement. It is all meant to adhere to an interpretive perspective in which risk-taking is understood as an expressive form—as an activity that embodies self and interpersonal relations, as experimental and future oriented, as deep play and *experience*.

PLAY AND TRANSFORMATIVE EXPERIENCE

The teenager who speaks of risks as if they were evidence of being a "participant," and the one who argues that risks have a role to play in growing up, are formulating an interpretation of risk as dramatic and transformative experience. The ubiquity of this interpretation was suggested in responses to the very first question, "What's the difference between something that risky and something that's not risky?" Virtually all of them reflected the idea of exploring new territory. Approximately 25% of the responses indicated that risks are different from nonrisks because they provide challenging or novel experiences; 65% emphasized the possibility of unknown or unintended consequences; the remaining 10% indicated that risks, more than nonrisks, have positive implications for peer relationships—friends are impressed by those who attempt the extraordinary.

The pioneering quality that separates risk from nonrisk was also reported to be the source of its appeal. Consider the following description of a physical risk that involved climbing a building whose architecture includes a series of ledges, diminishing in width so as to present an increasingly greater challenge to the climber:

> "What's fun is finishing it, getting done and saying, 'Hey, I walked all around it.' Because I'm sure there are some people who can't do it. I can say, 'Have you walked around the music building?', and they say, 'No.' 'Well, you should try it.' They

come a week later and say, 'I tried to and couldn't do it—I don't see how you can do it!' "

Risks were described as targets of astonishment and admiration not only for one's friends, but for oneself. When asked, "What's appealing about taking risks?" all of the teenagers referred to the pleasure or excitement in changing the status quo. Approximately 30% of the reasons they provided indicated that risks are appealing because of their developmental implications—they provide opportunities for learning about oneself and one's abilities. For example, "You want to see if you can do this new thing"; "doing what you're not sure of—that's what makes it exciting"; "it's a way of learning about life." Said another:

> "More and more my risk-taking is a conscious effort at experience and growth. I'm thinking ahead more of how it's going to help me in terms of experience. I want to reach out and touch as many things as I can. I'm kind of afraid that this life is too short to be content with what is easy to attain. It's better to reach out now when you have so much less responsibility— when you have the opportunity to reach out, take it."

Other responses cast risk's novelty in hydraulic terms, describing its ability to modulate levels of arousal and excitement (40%), or release tension (5%). Those few responses that referred to tension release also included explicit references to drug use. For example:

> "It's a release. When you're all together, it makes you feel good—makes things a lot more interesting and brings out the wild side of us. Last Friday we dropped acid. It gives you a different perspective on things. At school you have to be straight and set your mind on something but when you are free on a Friday night with your closest friends you can get wild and uninhibited, and getting fucked up has a lot to do with that. It's a way to relate—a different way of being close."

In this excerpt, it is apparent that the "release" has implications beyond a simple venting of frustrations or anxieties accumulated in more structured or demanding settings. Getting a "different perspective on things," getting "wild and uninhibited," not only makes you feel good, but provides for a different sort of interpersonal experience, a different sort of closeness. Several other responses (15%) focused more generally on the social implications of risks: They impress friends; they create shared memories; they give you something to talk and laugh about later. The remaining responses (10%) indicated that risks are appealing because they constitute an act of defiance and rebellion. Here, the possibility of "getting caught," or as one teenager aptly put it, "almost, but not quite getting caught," is a source of fun and excitement:

> "Doing something and getting away with it—it's a way of having fun. Or maybe the humor of it. You're driving at 80 miles per hour and stop at a stop sign and a cop will turn around the corner, and you start giggling. Or you're out drinking, or maybe you just smoked a joint, and you're walking downtown and say 'hi' to a police officer and he walks on by. It's trying to outsmart the older generation—trying to prove we're smarter. We're not, but we like to think we are."

The fun and playful nature of risks was discussed throughout the interviews, and associated often with the duping of authority:

> "Last night me and Michael went to this benefit concert at the school. It cost $10. I didn't want to pay to see a bunch of local bands, so we thought about sneaking in, but there were too many cops. But then when we were driving home we saw this car in this parking lot, which is on the other side of the school. And we recognized Mr. Gromley's car, who is this teacher who is real obnoxious and ultra-conservative. So we decided to roll his car. So we drove to the store and bought a bunch of toilet paper and came back, and started rolling the car. And a car drove right by us and we acted like we were taking the paper off. So when we were leaving, the attendant lady asked us what we were doing. We told her we were listening to the concert from over there."

Little deceptions often require well-laid plans, some of which were highly creative. One group of friends, for example, intended to sneak out one night, and made up the excuse that they wanted to wash the only available car—a Volkswagen—at the end of the street so as not to make a mess in front of the house. Naturally, they "didn't bother" to repark it, and were thus able to sneak quietly away in the middle of the night. Other strategies, however functional, or perhaps because they were functional, seemed ready-made, historically speaking. The most common and frequently cited example is the spending-the-night-at-a-friend's-house loop: Ellen is at Chelsea's is at Ellen's. Either way, sneaking out presents a challenge:

> "You have to plan ahead a lot. Last time, my friend spent the night with me. We put clothes in the bed [to resemble a body], and my boyfriend and his friends picked us up at the end of the block. We went to this friend's house who lives out in the country. Nothing really bad happened. There was a little drinking but no drugs that I knew about. There was loud music and dancing."

Sometimes the duping of authority is entirely unintended, and makes for great storytelling on that score alone:

> "I went to a party and everyone was drunk. There were some friends of my boyfriend and they wanted to go to Burger King, but they were too drunk to drive. But when they saw me they said, 'This is great!' and we all piled in the car, and I turned around and saw that they all had beer in the car. I think they were too far gone to notice. But it was one of those things—they were friends of my boyfriend—and I couldn't say, 'This is stupid, guys.' So I figured, 'It's only to Burger King,' so I took them. But on the way over they started arguing about how much clearance there was under the car, so this guy who is 3 months short of his 21st birthday jumps out of the car with his beer bottle to measure the distance. It's a stop light and there's no one around and I thought, 'Okay,' so he jumps back in the car and another car pulls up behind me. Of course it's a cop and he pulls us over. I didn't have my license because I left my purse at the party 'cuz it was just to Burger King. So the cop says, 'I saw you pull over and pick up a beer bottle.' The funny part is that he didn't think anybody in the car had been drinking, and they couldn't find my license number because he kept spelling my last name wrong, so he said, 'I'm sorry, but one of the other people in the car will have to drive.' I still can't believe it. The cop made one of the drunk guys drive us home."

The cop plays the fool in this story, and this is what makes it funny. But in this instance he was not forced into the role through the guts and guile of adolescent strategists. It just happened that way, as it did here:

> "We don't always 'decide' to do something risky. Sometimes it sort of just happens. When we were younger we would plan it, like putting shaving cream on someone's car, but now we don't always plan ahead. Like 2 weeks ago we were smoking pot in the back of my car. And this cop drove behind us and had his sirens on. So we tried to put up the dope and the cop just passed us. So we were real lucky then. But then we turned around and saw the cop turn around. So we hauled and went through lights and stuff and the cop never got us. It was a blast; scared the shit out of us."

It is noteworthy that pot-smoking in and of itself was less a risk than a catalyst for a car chase scene, the latter carrying the greater portion of interest. Indeed, the teenagers provided several other examples suggesting that getting high or drunk was little more than an admission ticket to an adolescent playground or amusement park. The excerpt that follows suggests that this is so. Equally noteworthy, however, is the suggestion that getting high or drunk was once, at a younger age, an end in itself:

> "In junior high school the risks were more obvious things like vandalism and smoking in the bathrooms because you couldn't smoke on campus then. Now it's a different attitude. You're still taking risks, but you aren't so blatant about it. It's not that you're trying to prove something to someone else. It's more spontaneous and not to get back at someone. Kids used to do it because they were tired of their parents or tired of the school rules. Now it's more to make people laugh. It's for fun or amusement and doesn't have that vindictive edge. It just comes with what you are doing, not so much on purpose. It used to be like that, like 'Let's go smoke some marijuana or drive recklessly and try to prove something by it.' Now it's if we do happen to be somewhere, we might think it would be fun to smoke some pot and do donuts in the parking lot, but it would not be planned."

Suggested here is a transition from an earlier period in which risky behaviors are goal objects consciously indulged and sought after—getting high, driving fast, going to wild parties. Later, however, goals become means, ways of creating or defining a "play space." This is expressed in the following reflection on the difference between "stupid risks" and those that carry a greater meaning because they are framed as play:

> "Some risks are meaningless and stupid, and some are meaningful. A meaningful risk would be like . . . it could be stupid, like pissing on a cop's car, but meaningful because probably everybody was drunk and it seemed really fun and it still is. A lot of the risk we do is when people are drunk. A meaningless risk would be like something stupid when you weren't drunk. Like if you pissed on a cop's car when you weren't drunk it would be really stupid—no one would think it was funny."

The bite is a nip; the blink is a wink; this is play. The duality of play, as elaborated in Chapter 4, defines a transitional space, a me and not-me:

> "I take risks just to see what it's like, just to do something, and because my friends are. [Drinking and partying is] something we're all doing together, and then everyone's really funny. It's to be together and not worry too much about what you're doing in front of these people. You can do outrageous things because you're drunk, which is awful. It shouldn't be like that, but that's the way it is."

Another made the telling point that getting drunk is "a good excuse to fall all over that cute guy you really like." According to Winnicott (1971), in a supportive, secure, and "facilitating" environment, the baby is never challenged about its transitional object. It is never made to answer the question: Did you create that or did you find it? (p. 89). Likewise, among friends, the adolescent will not be made to answer to the question: Was that your *real* self, or were you just *acting* that way because you were drunk?

In their definitions of risk, and their reflections on its appeal, the teenagers emphasized play and novelty, not for its own sake, but for its transformative power. It sets in motion a process nearly alchemical, one that can alter mental and emotional states, change one's interpersonal relationships or social status, or provide learning experiences. Many spoke of pushing personal limits, of feeling accomplished, of learning about life and responsibility. Said one, "It gives you inner strength and you can go on to try other things"; and another, "It proves something to your self—that you can do it."

> "It's sort of getting independence, and also something to look back on. Monday, at school, you can talk about all the crazy things you did over the weekend. But it's also like trying to grow up. Deep down inside you think that people will respect you more for it—the fact that you got away with it and didn't get caught. If you get caught, it can affect you for a long time. I have friends who have been caught and their parents don't trust them so they're really strict. You could also hurt someone, or hurt yourself, or cause embarrassment to yourself, like, 'There's another asshole teenager running around.' As long as you don't hurt anybody, or make anybody mad, and show respect for the older people. They can recognize quicker than you if you're acting like an asshole."

Several illustrated their points with personal stories, this provided by a 17-year-old girl:

> "The most recent risk was when I had about 15 people over when my parents were out of town for the weekend. That was really scary. I was afraid I was going to get caught. It was so fun. Parents make such a big deal out of leaving you at home and I guess my parents were scared I was going to have a party and trash the whole house. But it's just kind of exciting to know that I can get away with it without them knowing. But the house didn't get trashed and everyone was really responsible and I felt kind of old being able to pull off something like that. I invited only my closest friends and I told them that if there was going to be drinking that they are not going to drive and if they spend the night nothing [i.e., sex] happens. I made sure that the word didn't get out to anyone else and I made sure that there were only a few cars there. It was irresponsible to have it in the first place, but the way I handled it was responsible."

Most of the issues raised by the teenagers in reflecting on risks and their appeal have been captured within this particular story: the excitement of the novel or forbidden, the importance of achieving control over the unknown or unpredictable, feelings of responsibility and maturity that come from a risk well taken.

In tying their risks, and indeed their very development, to issues of exploration, control, and mastery, the teenagers reconstructed our cultural narrative of adolescence. In our culture, adolescence is considered a time of cognitive, emotional, and social upheaval. Individuals tossed about by these revolutionary forces are expected to take risks. Two individuals, both girls, explicitly linked adolescent risk-taking to depression. According to one:

> "Teens are less careful about their lives because it's the stereotypic thing with teenagers that, 'Oh, I hate my life.' I find that to be very true. For a lot of teenagers it's the cool thing to be really depressed, and that's how it transfers over to risks."

The other used similar terms to account for adolescent drinking: "They're more depressed, or think they are."

There are two points to be emphasized here. One is that many risk activities are symbolic of what it means to be an adolescent. The second is that part of being an adolescent involves a struggle to be someone more mature, and that by taking risks—drinking, smoking, curfew violations—teenagers involve themselves in activities that are largely symbolic of what it means to be adult (Jessor, 1987; Jessor & Jessor, 1975; Stacey & Davies, 1970).

TIME, EXPERIENCE, AND CULTURAL NARRATIVES

There is a sense, then, that risks are organized into a narrative structure in which they are linked with cultural concepts of development and the timing of life experiences. Within this structure, risks attain a degree of coherency—they are meaningful, intelligible. One of the primary functions of narrative forms is to structure events in such a way as to generate coherence and direction over time. In their analysis of life histories, the Gergens (1983) identified three rudimentary forms of narrative that can be mapped onto the intersecting dimensions of "evaluation" and "time," as shown in Figure

5.1. One form, the "stability narrative" (Part A in Figure 5.1), links events over time in a way that leaves the individual essentially unchanged. For example, "My work continues to go well and successfully" (N1), or "I still can't make it in the major league" (N2). The two other narrative forms (Part B in Figure 5.1), one "progressive," one "regressive," are linked with the production of positive or negative change. In the progressive case, for example, "I've overcome a lot of obstacles to get where I am today" (N1). Or, in the regressive case, "I just can't seem to get a handle on the issues anymore" (N2).

The Gergens' analysis is easily transported to the teenagers' discussions of risk involvement. Even risks gone awry were consid-

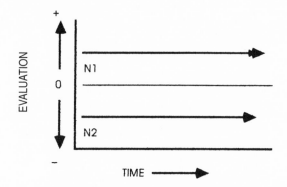

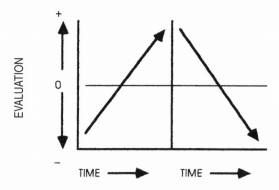

FIGURE 5.1. Three narrative forms.

ered instruments of positive growth, learning, and development—recall the young man who claimed that the appeal of risk-taking lies in the potential for inner growth, independence, and maturity, and that "even if I fail, I still kind of pat myself on the back and say, 'Hey, you tried it, and no one can blame you for sitting back and not participating.'"

Valsiner (1994b) has likened narrative forms to cultural tools that canalize thinking and reasoning about past events. He notes, however, that narrative constructions are not undertaken for the purpose of reliving the past, or recounting it in veridical terms. Rather, the past is recollected, organized, and justified in anticipation of things to come, of what might be—in anticipation, that is, of some hypothetical and imagined point of view (see also Schiebe, 1986).

That adolescent risk-taking is given meaning and made coherent in light of a partially unknown, although nonetheless tangible, future was particularly apparent in discussions of how their risks would change as they matured. Only (15%) provided a stability narrative, arguing that their risks would not change because they themselves would not change; they would have the "same priorities," "values," or the same desire to "avoid boredom." All of the others indicated that their involvement in risks would change over time in a manner consistent with general and normative developments. Of these, only 10% were regressive narratives, in which a decline in risk activities was linked to declining physical abilities—their bodies, quite simply, would become incapable of tolerating the risks' abuse. The vast majority, however, produced progressive narratives consistent with our cultural conceptions of development as a movement toward increasing abilities, competencies, opportunities, and sophistication. For a few (15%), risks were expected to increase, especially in college, because there would be more opportunities to take them (i.e., less adult supervision). But most expected to take fewer risks as they matured. Some made reference to cognitive advancements, and claimed that risks would decline with increased knowledge of negative outcomes. Others referred to a change in legal status. Alcohol consumption, for example, would no longer be illegal and therefore not risky. General experience was also considered relevant, as risks taken during adolescence lost their potency to excite and challenge. These developments notwithstanding, the most frequent explanation for the anticipated decline concerned changes in duties and responsibilities that accompany adulthood, changes that would preclude opportunities or diminish the willingness to engage in risky practices.

> "I think my risk-taking will change as I get older. I think [we'll take fewer risks] after we get it out of our system and really experience more about the bad things that can happen. I think everyone changes. What is fun now will not be fun for us in 5 years. Also, there will be more responsibilities, and other things become fun. Probably take more sensible risks, I would think, and it wouldn't be for fun anymore. It would be life-relating kinds of things, like maybe at a job."

> ["Will your risk-taking change as you get older?"] "I hope so. I don't want to go to college the way I am. I'm sure I could induce a change if I tried, but at the moment I'm still in high school having fun, and I don't really want to change. In college I'll have to be a little more mature because I'll be living my own life; I'll have to accept responsibility."

> "When you're older you get more set in your ways, and if you were to mess up on this one thing it would really affect you. Right now it wouldn't have much effect, but if you were older it could affect your way of life in a certain way. You'd have, like, a family. Now you have a family but you are their responsibility. If you got hurt, they'd help you out. If you got older and you got hurt and you're supposed to look after other people, but you'd need them to look after you."

Thus, the majority of the teenagers provided progressive narratives, but in all cases the change (or stability) in risk involvement was linked to anticipated developments of the future. Typically, these developments were expected to suppress risk behaviors: The teenagers would become more competent in evaluating the potential outcomes of their actions; they would mature physically (albeit in a degenerative fashion); their legal status would change; but mostly, socially prescribed role expectations would dictate more conservative behavior. As one individual explained, "I have the excuse of being a teenager now—I don't have many responsibilities." Another described adolescent recklessness and irresponsibility as a character trait:

"The teenage mentality is one of carelessness. Part of being a teen is you don't have much responsibility as you will have later. You're irresponsible because in other situations you're allowed to be. It carries over. It gets into people's personalities."

The idea that risks are an adolescent affair soon to be upstaged by responsibilities of work and family is expressed succinctly here:

"I think in college I will take more risks just because it is a different situation and I will be meeting more people and have more opportunities to do things. I guess when I get older and if I get married then I'll try to set a good example for the kids. When you have children you can't always bring them along. There are just not many opportunities. And once you get in that frame of mind, when the opportunity does come up, you wouldn't be as prepared to take it because you've been holding out for so long."

Another individual also spoke of age-graded social expectations:

"People don't take many risks after college. You have to set an example for society when you're that age. If you're a teenager and get drunk every weekend, it's all right. But if you're an adult and it gets around the neighborhood it doesn't look good. Instead of looking like a normal teenager, you look like a drunkard. You have to conform to what's expected."

Adolescents' understanding that their risk involvement takes place against the backdrop of culturally prescribed role expectations was also borne out in their predictions of who would get more drunk at a New Year's Eve party, a teenager or a parent. Only one thought that both would get equally drunk. Three more thought that the parent would get more drunk because adults set aside special occasions for such behavior, and New Year's Eve is one of them. The remaining participants nominated the teenager as the more likely candidate. Some fairly typical responses include the following:

"A lot of teenagers get really drunk as opposed to grownups who drink less. The kids don't have alcohol available to them all the time and so they would take advantage of it. None of my friends drink for the pleasure of it, like a glass of wine or something like my dad at dinner. When they drink it would be to get drunk. When you are at a party and you feel kind of strange, you feel like the party hasn't really gotten started. There will be a lot of people there but nothing really happens so you drink and then you loosen up and then it gives you an excuse to do stupid things."

"The kid would get drunker. My parents go out and drink socially. On New Year's Eve and being a teenager and you have access to that kind of stuff, it's like, 'Let's bring in the New Year with a bang.' And also, it's like the forbidden fruit. It's a lot of fun and we are not suppose to do this. New Year's for adults might be depressing: 'Oh, no! Another year!'"

"Paula [or Paul; the character's name was kept consitent with the gender of the respondent] will get more drunk because the mother has more responsibility and can handle the peer pressure better. She doesn't have a bunch of rowdy friends. With teenagers, it's accepted to get drunk. They want to be like their other friends, and act cool to impress each other."

"At a high school party it's real normal to get really drunk. But to get real drunk at an adults' party—I can see the adults looking at him [Paul's father] like, 'You drunkard.' So the dad wouldn't get so drunk. With teenagers, it's accepted by their peers. If you see an adult get drunk at a party you think it's his personality where he's drunk all the time, but if you're a kid and you get drunk every weekend it's just accepted. Kids don't see it as a permanent problem. It's a temporary thing."

By and large, their reasons fit the following descriptors:

◆ Drinking is a means of defying authority (10%).
◆ Getting drunk is still novel and exciting (30%).
◆ The teenager is still uncertain about how much alcohol is "too much" alcohol, and will err inevitably on the side of excess (15%).
◆ The teenager will conform to the social expectation that adolescents drink more than adults, or drink for the purpose of becoming intoxicated, that is, "the feeling rather than the taste" (35%)

◆ The teenager will be inclined to use alcohol for the purpose of feeling more comfortable in social interactions, or as an "excuse" for engaging in potentially unacceptable behavior; for example, "It's a good excuse to fall all over that cute guy you really like" (10%).

Clearly, the teenagers' interpretations of risk involvement drew heavily from cultural conceptions of adolescence, and expressed a particular epistemology regarding the relationship between experience and development. Risks are understood to chart a course for personal growth and social relationships, and the course runs especially deep and true for those on the cusp of maturity. "The friends you have as a teenager are the best you'll ever have because you're allowed by society to have fun"; "After you have a family—well, it's not like you have to impress your wife all the time."

SOCIAL POSITIONING AND MORALLY CONTROVERSIAL LEISURE

The structure, organization, or interpretation of adolescent risk-taking is not a cultural narrative that was copied, appropriated, or borrowed wholesale for the functional purpose of imposing meaning on one's experience. There was a sense, instead, that adolescents considered their experiences instrumental to creating those meanings. Here, a teenager expresses his understanding about how shared risks strengthen interpersonal ties, and also reawaken the bonds of friendship once the risks themselves have been outworn:

"My two best friends graduated, so I don't do as much anymore. We'd go swimming in the lake in the middle of winter, race our cars around on some of the back roads, sometimes get pretty destructive. It was fun, but now I'm calming down. I'm not as inclined to do it alone. It would be lonely. It kind of strengthens the bond of friendship. If it's something risky then you'll both remember it fondly, having outgrown it. You think back to the time you drove the car at 90 mph and hit a speed bump and took off in the air. It was kind of scary—you remember who was in the car with you."

Risks were seen to occupy a privileged role in development largely because of the meaning they carry and what they communicate to others. Even the young man who spoke of inner growth and internal feelings of independence and maturity made reference to someone, perhaps only himself, who might blame him for sitting back and not participating. Harré and van Langenhove (1991) have argued that social actions, from the simplest conversations to the most complex institutional practices, involve a sort of posturing in which one's identity is collected, expressed, and positioned in relation to others. Bakhtin (1981) has pointed out, however, that not all social action is equally self-demonstrative. Business memos, for example, belong to a genre that can reflect only the most superficial aspects of self. Genres that are most conducive to self-expression, or self-conscious social positioning, are artistic and aesthetic; self-expression, in fact, is their main goal.

More than most other forms of social action, adolescents' risk involvement necessarily entails a self-conscious positioning on the part of participants because of its deviant status. Adults define what is sensible or irrational, what is morally appropriate or offensive. They define the boundaries, in other words, between what is acceptable and what is deviant. Adolescents bent on crossing these boundaries must make provisions to protect their activities from disruptions: They become secretive, withdraw to secluded areas, close themselves off from those who will not participate. Gary Alan Fine (1992) referred to such activity as "morally controversial leisure" and argued that it requires a reflective awareness because of the rhetoric of justification needed to defend the activity, to deflect attacks, to claim a moral high ground. Bakhtin (1981) said as much when he distinguished between a prior, acknowledged, *authoritative discourse* and an emerging, experimental, *internally persuasive discourse*, the latter being of decisive significance in the evolution of consciousness. He argued that the process of distinguishing between one's own discourse and that of another is activated rather late in development, and wrote that "[w]hen thought begins to work in an independent, experimenting and discriminating way, what first occurs is a separation between internally persuasive discourse and authoritarian enforced discourse, along with a rejection of those congeries of discourses that do not matter to us, that do not touch us"

(p. 345). The process by which this is accomplished is semiotic. Discourses are objectified and positioned in text, a process, he said, that "becomes especially important when someone is striving to liberate himself from the influence of such an image and its discourse. . . . The importance of struggling with an other's discourse, its influence in the history of an individual's coming to ideological consciousness, is enormous" (p. 348).

The extent to which adolescents' risks represent a struggle between these categories of discourse is expressed in the following:

> "I feel very close to my brother, but I don't really like my mom or dad. My mom's trying to hold me down a lot. She's very overprotective with me and my brother. She makes me want to get the hell out of here more and get away from her. It just makes me want to try all sorts of stuff—to see what my limitations are. So *I* can know what I can do, rather than my mom saying what abilities you have and don't have and what you can do with your life. I feel like it's mine. It's up to me to find out what I can do mentally and physically."

As a note of reassurance, most of the adolescents interviewed appeared to like and respect their parents. Nevertheless, they were emphatic in their desires to separate themselves, their activities, their interests and knowledge from their parents:

> "It's hard for me to have a group of friends and my mom there. She works with young kids and she's really good at reading people, and I have a problem with her trying to be my friends' friend. I like my mom, but she tries to talk to my friends like a friend. She wants to find out more about them and I feel like she is always watching me. Not to be nosy so much; just because she's interested in my life. It really bothers me."

Although adolescents' risk-taking can be construed in terms of a struggle with the authoritative discourse of another, it is also a mechanism for creating a discourse of their own, the internally persuasive one that Bakhtin wrote of. By these lights, the reflective awareness that is engendered, the coming into ideological consciousness that follows in the wake of such struggle, is coupled dialectically to processes of sociocultural identification. Untanglings and entanglements; engagement with another's point of view is the fountainhead of mindedness.

STRUCTURE AND CONSTRAINTS

There is nothing as emancipating as a good constraint: This point has been made by Winegar, Renninger, and Valsiner (1989) in the course of developing the concept of "dependent-independence" (see also Renninger & Winegar, 1985). With it, they mean to move beyond a view of development in which the child progresses from a state of dependence upon its environment and those within it, to one of autonomy and independence. Specifically, they retire the notion that dependence and independence are polar opposites, and define them, instead, as aspects of a unified whole. Children become increasingly competent, responsible, and "independent" within a context of dependence on others who provide "differential constraints" in the service of "progressive empowerment." The gist of the argument is that the structuring and organization of mental life is unavoidably linked to the structuring and organization of social action and culture. In this regard, the concept is similar in attitude to that of inclusive separation. Psychic and social realities, although distinct, are conjoined and take their form within a process of participation. A suggestion of this process is apparent in the following excerpt provided by an individual who felt already the yoke of impending responsibility in sufficient degree as to alter his previous patterns of risk-taking. We see in this instance a complex interweaving of changing legal sanctions, parental constraints, and personal experience, all of which coalesce in an understanding of the implications of actions:

> "I've had it with my wild and crazy days. They mess you up. Now I have to plan for the future. Sometimes my friends say I've become chicken, but if there are too many bad things that can go on . . . I want to know all the consequences of something before I do it—all the possibilities and the worst that can happen. Now that I'm 16, everything goes on my record. I guess it's responsibilities put on me. I have to get good grades

or I'll lose my license. I have to think of the future. I like to stay in control. I don't like getting out of control because everything comes down on you. I wouldn't take a risk where I lose control. And there's a difference between drugs and alcohol. I've already had my experience with pot and it messes me up. So now I'm really scared of that, and at parties if I see it I just go into another room. And pot and drugs are illegal for everyone where alcohol is only illegal by age. I can see my limit on risk-taking. I found the line by experimenting. I started in ninth grade. I'm trying to get an understanding with my parents that instead of sneaking out like I used to, that they let me stay out a little later—30 minutes later."

The teenagers often brought up this more or less explicit negotiation of risk and responsibility that takes place between themselves and their parents. I recall in this context a conversation with an individual who summarized a lecture delivered recently by his father. The topic concerned the difference between trouble with a "little t" and trouble with a "big T." Although the former is still trouble, and weighted with unhappy consequences, it is to some extent expected and tolerated. The consequence for trouble of the latter sort, on the other hand, is a monster under the bed—chthonian, inscrutable, and doubtlessly dangerous:

"This house is easy to get out of. I can get out any time I want to: late at night, early in the morning. Sometimes they know, but as long as I don't do anything. . . . The first time I got caught, I went out one night and stayed out late and my mom heard me come back and told me to tell Dad before she did. I went up to him and told him and he said, 'There's little t and big T'—It's a speech I'll remember for a long time—'As long as you keep in the little t category and keep it cool and it's not something that's serious, I'll be bearable to live with. But don't push your luck. If you get into big T, it will be BIG T, and you will be in serious stuff.' Like getting drunk: Well, drunk isn't a good word for it. I'll just say that I know what beer tastes like. I've never had an uncontrollable feeling. Well, I shouldn't say that because I have, but we always designate a driver. We always will. We sat down and talked about it. We're not going to get into the kind of trouble we've seen other kids get in."

I bring this up to demonstrate how risks are construed as a means of crossing certain boundaries and sampling new experiences, but are nonetheless socially organized, limited, and channeled. Some boundaries are relatively universal in middle-class America: Adolescents are not permitted to use drugs or alcohol, to skip school, to have sexual intercourse. These boundaries define novel domains of experience, many of which, as argued previously, are symbols of maturity. There are also historical, cultural, and familial differences in adolescents' understanding of how their behavior is organized, and we would expect to see these differences expressed in risk behaviors. For example, diaries written by young men of the 17th century indicate that sneaking out of the house in the middle of the night was probably as common then as it is now. Although this particular risk spans historical time in conjunction with the curfew, 17th-century youths used their unsupervised moments to play cards with their friends, an activity frowned upon by clergy and good families alike. We would be hard pressed, I think, to find this particular form of risk exhibited by today's teenagers.

PARENTAL CONSTRAINTS: A COMPARATIVE ANALYSIS

The manner by which risks are related to adolescents' perceptions of how their behavior is constrained is seen more fully in a comparative analysis of two teenagers whose family backgrounds differed markedly. The first case is that of a 16-year-old boy who dropped out of high school in the middle of his sophomore year. His parents set few limits on his behavior, and he reported that he can "come and go" as he pleased: "That's the way it is between me and my parents." Although he was not in school, neither was he employed; his activities were relatively unconstrained. The boy indicated that he differs from his friends because, as he said,

> "I don't think I *should* do anything, or I *can't* do anything. They [friends] want to have things that they should do and things they can and can't do. I don't think there's anything I should or shouldn't do. ["Where do your friends get these ideas about what they should and shouldn't do?"] I guess from themselves and their parents and everyone else they are around."

Not only does this teenager feel that his action possibilities are unlimited, his interpersonal relationships also appear to lack cohesiveness. He claimed that he has no close friends, and that "I don't think of me and my friends as a group; the main reason we are together is because we get along and we like to smoke marijuana." (I should mention that the other members of this group [discussed more fully in Chapter 6] reported a great deal of interpersonal closeness.)

Without boundaries to provide at least some minimal definition of risk and nonrisk (much less sort through risks with *big T* or *little t* consequences), we might expect that this teenager would find little appeal in risk-taking. This was apparent in the interview. A personal story illustrates the point:

> "We were sneaking out almost every night when we had something to smoke. I don't have to sneak out, I can just leave. But my friends really have to sneak out, so maybe it's exciting for them, but it's a pain for me. If I'm driving that night I have to wait 3 hours and I'll want to do it right then [smoke the marijuana], but I have to wait and it's a huge hassle. I'd rather do it during the day because there's less hassle."

Perhaps a more dramatic illustration of the relationship between perceived boundaries and the excitement of moving beyond them is provided in his description of getting a drivers' license. Not being able to drive was one of the few limits places on his behavior. In contrast to every other adolescent interviewed who reported a blissful freedom in getting a license, this particular teenager resented it. In his words:

> "It spoils things. Before I started driving I was a lot closer to my friends. It was a big thing to go over to each other's houses. You couldn't just drive over there and say 'hi' and leave. But now we'll stop by each other's houses and its just so casual that it's just too cool."

Thus, the absence of effort was associated with a lack of commitment. This individual has difficulty understanding how his behavior, his interpersonal relationships, and indeed, his future, are organized and thus given meaning. There are no transforming experiences for him; no real *experience* at all. No learning by trying and erring, because there is no trying. He does "what comes naturally," his words apropos of Vygotsky's (1979) distinction between natural, knee-jerk behaviors, and higher, "cultural" actions by which we structure, experience, understand, and control our lives. This individual who could come and go as he pleased; who had several times dropped out of school; who was a frequent user of alcohol, pot, and hallucinogens; and who had several contacts with police for minor and sundry infractions, argued that these weren't risks, really, and he wasn't much of a risk-taker. As improbable as that sounds on the face of it, I think he's right. He summarized his situation as follows:

> "As I get older I feel that I've been wasting time long enough and it's time to get serious, even though I'm a high school dropout. But I'm not in control of my life now. I'm not happy with my situation."

In stark contrast to the case just presented, this story concerns a 16-year-old girl whose parents were perceived as highly controlling. When asked about her friends and what they did together, she related what she called her "family history":

> "My mom especially is real insecure and protective and paranoid that everything bad in the world is going to happen if she lets me do anything. So up until this summer I have never even gone to the movies with a friend. I have never hung out with friends. It's just never been a part of my life."

What does one do in a situation where constraints are highly explicit and strictly enforced, with no opportunities to move beyond them? This young woman adopted a "strategy" of fantasizing risks. She went so far as to describe it as "rebelliousness," and so it was:

> "Rebelling isn't very fun. You can end up getting caught like I did. I had a diary and wrote down everything I thought—who I liked at the time, how I felt about them. They are the kinds of things you don't write down if you think someone is going to read them. And someone read them. I'd write down who I

talked to on the phone and what I said and it would be a boy [she was not allowed telephone conversations with boys]. And they read it and thought I was going to turn out to be some kind of a smutty person. They lost all trust in me. And it was the year of my confirmation in church. And they were, like, 'I don't think you should be confirmed; I don't think you care about God at all.' They thought I was a really bad kind of person. I knew I wasn't. I knew that I had just written down what I was thinking, that I wasn't going to act on what I thought ["What kinds of things?"] Like, 'I think he likes me.' I was grounded for 2 months—no radio, no phone, or anything. What's funny for me is that grounding isn't a punishment because I could never do anything in the first place."

This teenager's fantasies appear remarkably similar to risks taken in "real time" by her peers: They were construed as a form of rebellion, and "getting caught" carried negative consequences. Her case is also interesting because in spite of severe restrictions imposed by her parents, she felt that much of her behavior was self-determined:

"I don't have time to hang out with friends. I'm too busy. And the reason I'm so cautious against taking risks is that I work at school and the kinds of grades I get is really, really important to me because I want to go to medical school at Harvard. It's incredibly hard to keep a 4.0 in high school."

Her appraisal invites speculation. It is clearly at odds with earlier comments—a defense, perhaps, but one that keeps her focused in a domain in which she has chosen to excel through efforts of her own. In this, her situation seems more hopeful than that of the young man who is "not in control," who has been "wasting time," and needs to "get serious." In reflecting on her family circumstances and where they might lead, she discussed her sister, who had gone to college the previous year and jeopardized her status there by "going wild." The teenager that I interviewed recognized the difficulty in moving to college from a closed and rigid family environment that restricted opportunities for making decisions, having choices, and taking chances. She hoped that she would do better than her sister.

BOYS AND GIRLS

In addition to the constraints of family, as above, gender categories were also found to be relevant to the teenagers' interpretations of risk involvement. The Risk and Adventure Checklist was given in paper-and-pencil format, and was designed to elicit preferences for novel experiences under different conditions. As shown in Table 5.1, it included several sets of personally descriptive propositions, each

TABLE 5.1. Risk and Adventure Checklist Items

Item 1.	I like to do new things *a.* just to see what happens *b.* only when I'm fairly sure about what will happen *c.* that I know I can do easily
Item 2.	When my friends and I are looking for fun *a.* I try to get them to do something none of us has done before *b.* I'm easily persuaded to do something that one of them likes, but that I've never done before *c.* I try to get them to do something that I like and have done before
Item 3.	I get a feeling of accomplishment when *a.* I do something really wild and succeed *b.* I do somthing that's challenging but somewhat familiar *c.* I succeed at things I've done in the past
Item 4.	Once I've decided to do something new *a.* I plunge in wholeheartedly *b.* I try to prepare for the sonsequences *c.* I worry a lot about what might happen

Items 5 and 6. I feel closer to a (same-sex/opposite-sex) friend when we do something together that
  a. neither of us has done before
  b. he/she has done before, but is new for me
  c. that I've done before, but is new for him/her

Items 7 and 8. When I really want to get to know someone of the (same sex/opposite sex) better
  a. he/she can easily convince me to do something I've never done before
  b. I'm likely to ask him/her to do something with me that I think he/she has never done before.
  c. it's best to do something familiar together

set addressing a particular issue (e.g., feelings of accomplishment, getting to know someone of the opposite sex).

Each set contained three propositions, which the participants rank-ordered according to how well each expressed their personal preferences. The rank orders within each set were used to determine the individual's "pattern preference" for each issue. Regarding the issue of feeling accomplished (Item 3), for example, the rank order may indicate that *b* ("challenging but somewhat familiar") is preferred to *a* ("really wild and succeed") which is preferred to *c* ("done in the past"), that is, *b* > *a* > *c*.

Frequencies of pattern preferences are presented in Table 5.2. For Item 1, "I like to do new things," it can been seen that the most favored proposition was "just to see what happens." In contrast, "things that I know I can do easily" was least preferred. Overall, the adolescents indicated preferences for some degree of novelty. This was also the case for Item 2, although the pattern preferences were more evenly distributed. Thus, "When my friends and I are looking for fun," a preference for familiar activities, in the sense of getting friends "to do something I like and have done before," was not uncommon (more than 25% generated a pattern in which this proposition was the first choice). For Item 3, Patterns 1 and 2, which linked feelings of accomplishment with the "really wild" and "challenging" as opposed to the tried and true, were the most popular, accounting for nearly 50% of all responses. Responses to Item 4, "Once I've decided to try something new," showed that almost 50% of the

TABLE 5.2. Percentages of Pattern Preferences for Risk and Adventure Checklist

Pattern preference	Checklist item (N = 39)							
	1	2	3	4	5	6	7	8
1: *a* > *b* > *c*	41.0	30.8	46.2	28.2	38.5	23.1	12.8	10.3
2: *a* > *c* > *b*	7.3	5.1	2.6	2.6	33.3	35.9	12.8	17.9
3: *b* > *a* > *c*	17.9	17.9	38.5	25.6	12.8	17.9	7.7	12.8
4: *b* > *c* > *a*	23.1	17.9	5.1	23.1	0	2.6	12.8	12.8
5: *c* > *a* > *b*	0	5.1	0	2.6	0	12.8	17.9	17.9
6: *c* > *b* > *a*	7.7	20.5	2.6	17.9	12.8	7.7	30.8	17.9
Intransitive	2.6	2.6	5.1	0	2.6	0	5.1	10.3

teenagers try to anticipate consequences (i.e., Patterns 3 and 4 in which proposition *b* was the first choice), but more than 30% plunge in wholeheartedly (proposition *a*). In contrast, only 20% reported that they worry a lot about what might happen.

The remaining items (5–8) tapped into beliefs about the interpersonal contexts of sharing novel and familiar experiences. Items 5 and 6 asked about the role of such experiences in engendering feelings of closeness between same-sex friends (Item 5) and opposite-sex friends (Item 6). For Item 5 there was a clear preference for the first two patterns, in which the first choice was to feel closer to a same-sex friend by doing something that was novel for both self and friend. Novelty for both was also preferred for Item 6, which asked about feeling closer to an opposite-sex friend, although to a lesser extent. Item 7 focused on getting to know someone of the same sex, and responses were distributed somewhat more evenly here. However, almost 50% indicated a preference for Patterns 5 and 6, a preference, that is, for doing something familiar together. There was also a tendency (over 35%) to prefer the familiar in the case of getting to know someone of the opposite sex (Item 8).

In retrospect, it is unfortunate that the choices available for Items 5 and 6 (feeling closer to someone) were not comparable to those available for Items 7 and 8 (getting to know someone). That is, doing something novel for both was not included in the propositions for Items 7 and 8, nor was doing something familiar together an option for Items 5 and 6. It may be that the preferences for the familiar in the case of getting to know someone for and novelty in the case of feeling closer indicate that the value of different types of experiences is variable and subject to the developmental status of the relationship. Evidence for this argument will be presented in the next chapter. On the other hand, it may be that teenagers simply prefer to be on equal footing with their peers (novel *for both*, familiar *for both*), regardless of the nature of their relationships. Although this notion of experiential reciprocity has intuitive appeal, it is undermined somewhat in findings of gender differences, which suggest that the type of relationship (boy with girl or girl with boy) *does* matter.

Each item of the Checklist was analyzed for gender differences using the chi-square procedure. Interestingly, significant differences emerged only for those items addressing opposite-sex relationships

TABLE 5.3. Percentages of Boys' and Girls' Pattern Preferences on Items 6 and 8

Pattern preference	Item 6 (feel closer to opposite sex)		Item 8 (get to know opposite sex)	
	Boys ($N=21$)	Girls ($N=18$)	Boys ($N=19$)	Girls ($N=16$)
1: $a > b > c$	4.8	44.3	0	25.0
2: $a > c > b$	42.9	27.8	10.5	31.2
3: $b > a > c$	19.0	16.7	15.8	12.5
4: $b > c > a$	0	5.6	26.3	0
5: $c > a > b$	19.0	5.6	21.1	18.8
6: $c > b > a$	14.3	0	26.3	12.5

Note. The reported N's changed on Item 8 because intransitive responses were excluded.

(Items 6 and 8).[1] Pattern preferences for these two items are presented in Table 5.3, organized by gender.

Regarding Item 6, it can be seen that for most boys and girls, feeling closer to an opposite-sex friend was thought best accomplished by a joint activity that was new to both individuals (i.e., a preference for Patterns 1 and 2). On the other hand, there were clear gender differences for Pattern 1 versus Pattern 2, suggesting that the second best choice for accomplishing closeness is different for girls and boys. That is, girls, more than boys, were likely to choose Pattern 1 ("novel for both" preferred to "novel for me" preferred to "novel for him"), whereas boys were more likely to choose Pattern 2 ("novel for both" preferred to "novel for her" preferred to "novel for me"). This also held for Patterns 5 and 6: One-third of the boys chose these patterns in which closeness was best achieved by doing something that the girl has never done before, but was familiar to themselves. In contrast, only one girl indicated a preference for promoting closeness by sharing an experience familiar to her, but new to the boy. It would seem then, that the overall gender difference found for Item 6 may reflect boys' desires to introduce girls to something new, and girls' desires to be introduced by a boy

[1]The chi-square values and their corresponding p levels for Items 1 through 8, respectively, are as follows: $\chi^2 = 1.67$, $p = .90$; $\chi^2 = 6.17$, $p = .29$; $\chi^2 = 4.06$, $p = .60$; $\chi^2 = 5.36$, $p = .37$; $\chi^2 = 2.04$, $p = .85$; $\chi^2 = 12.37$, $p = .03$; $\chi^2 = 8.43$, $p = .13$; $\chi^2 = 11.74$, $p = .04$.

with experience. In fact, if preferences are summed across Patterns 1, 3, and 4 (in which "new for me" is preferred to "new for opposite-sex friend") and compared with the sum across Patterns 2, 5, and 6 (in which "new for friend" is preferred to "new for me"), we find reliable gender differences by the chi-square procedure. Specifically, as shown in Table 5.4, 76% of the boys, compared to 33% of the girls, chose patterns (2, 5, 6) in which "new for friend" was preferred to "new for me." All told, the analysis of Item 6 indicates that teenagers believe that heterosexual relationships will become more intimate when both members share a new experience, but failing that, boys ought to be on terra firma from which they can introduce girls to new activities, and both boys and girls believe in the importance of this asymmetry.

The analysis of Item 8, focused on getting to know someone of the opposite sex, tells essentially the same story. Returning to Table 5.3, we find that most girls (56%) chose Patterns 1 and 2, both of which indicate a first choice of engaging in an activity that they have never done before, as opposed to one that is new for the boy or familiar to both. In contrast, boys were more inclined to prefer activities that were new for the girl, or familiar to both. As with Item 6, preferences were summed across Patterns 1, 2, and 5 ("new for me" preferred to "new for friend") and 3, 4, and 6 ("new for friend" preferred to "new for me"). As shown in Table 5.4, nearly 70% of the boys, but only 25% of the girls, preferred patterns (3, 4, 6) in which

TABLE 5.4. Items 6 and 8 Reorganized: Percentages of Boys' and Girls' Pattern Preferences for "Novel for Friend" versus "Novel for Self"

Pattern preference	Boys	Girls
Item 6	($N = 21$)	($N = 18$)
Novel for friend	76.2	33.3
Novel for self	23.8	66.7
Item 8	($N = 19$)	($N = 16$)
Novel for friend	68.4	25.0
Novel for self	31.6	75.0

Note. The reported N's changed on Item 8 because intransitive responses were excluded.

the activity was familiar to themselves, but novel for the opposite-sex friend. The chi-square procedure indicated that these differences were reliable.

These findings are consistent with cultural stereotypes about men, women and adventure. Similar themes are played out in fairy tales: The young maiden is swept off her feet, or rescued from her captivity in a locked and lonely tower, or snatched from the jaws of a dragon, or woken from a dreamless sleep by some young adventurer who charges through the countryside building his reputation on such good works.

FRIENDSHIPS AND GROUP RELATIONS

Adolescents are in the process of forging identities in fellowship with their peers and, as argued previously, risks and adventures have a privileged role to play in this process. As "deep play" they disclose aspects of self and its relations. This is apparent in the following portion of the study, in which the participants were asked to speculate about the interpersonal consequences of sharing risks with close friends or acquaintances, and about how the consequences might vary according to the degree of risk involved (see also Lightfoot, 1992). The first scenario concerned a teenager who was offered a marijuana cigarette at a music concert:

> This is a story about a guy (girl) named Eric (Erica) who won four tickets from a local radio station to see a big-name rock band perform at the Smith Center. He asked three friends to go with him, and they were really excited because the concert had been sold out for weeks. They met at Eric's because his parents said he could use the car. After the car was parked in the stadium lot, one of the friends pulled a joint out of his sock. His older brother (sister) had given it to him to smoke before the concert. The friend lit the joint, and passed it to the other friends who each smoked some of it. Then it was passed to Eric. None of the friends had ever smoked pot before, and Eric felt a little unsure. Would Eric be more likely, less likely, or equally likely to smoke the pot with his *best* friends compared to friends who weren't as close? Why? If Eric smokes the pot with his best friends, will that affect how the friends think and feel about each other or not necessarily? Why? If Eric doesn't smoke the pot with his best friends, will

that affect how the friends think and feel about each other, or not necessarily? Why?

Nearly all of the teenagers (85%) argued that the story character would be more inclined to smoke with acquaintances compared to close friends. Reasons focused on the power of shared risks to transform different types of relationships: "It's a chance to impress them"; "To become part of their group"; "It's easy for friends who aren't close to form a bad opinion of you"; "Close friends look into the person, not the person's actions." Nonetheless, declining to participate in a risky activity, even in the company of close friends, places one on the outside of a shared experience, and if indulged too often, may threaten one's membership in the group. Several individuals (20%) noted that Eric could have provided reasonable justifications for his refusal (he had to drive), which would vitiate the negative consequences. A few even suggested that the responsibility of driving should rotate so that all can participate. Here are a few examples:

> "If his friends are doing it, and [he knows that] his brother does it, then he'll probably do it. He doesn't want to rain on their parade. You don't just think about yourself when you're with your friends. You're not self-centered. You think about if they have fun. And it will definitely bring them closer. Like a brotherhood—passing the test, the initiation, sharing a new experience and doing something totally new that you'll remember for quite a while. You remember who you're with. You can make an analogy with sex. The first person you have sex with you're going to be closer with because it's new and different"

> "He doesn't want these people who he doesn't know well to think that they don't like him. But if he's with his really good friends and decides not to, they're not going to hold it against him. With real good friends it wouldn't matter; with acquaintances it would. But he won't have as much fun because he'll be second guessing himself in his mind: 'Maybe I should have smoked it.'"

> "He's already established with best friends. He's secure there so he can relax more and focus more on what he wants. [If he doesn't smoke it] they could still have a lot of fun. The people who got stoned—their experience would be different than his,

so they may have bonded more with each other than with him, but that could be overcome. The people who got stoned would be closer. It's just like any other new experience. It would pull them together because it's a new thing—bonding."

It happened often that personal experiences were brought to bear on discussions of the hypothetical scenarios. The following account discloses the degree to which the developmental status of social relationships can organize an adolescent's willingness to engage in risky behavior:

> "I can be talked into the risk-taking stuff when I'm not really comfortable with the people I'm around. Then I'm bad about going ahead and giving in to peer pressure. Like driving with this friend of my sister's. I really didn't know him, but I certainly didn't feel safe driving with him. But there wasn't really a way to get out of the situation."

Her ambivalence is unmistakable, as is the recognition of her own poor judgment. Many of the individuals who were interviewed showed uncanny insight into the social processes and motivations of themselves and their friends:

> "People always look at getting high together as a sort of bonding experience, but I never see it that way. A good example is that I have heard these semi-friends talking, and I don't think they were that good of friends with themselves, but yet one of them was saying to the other, 'Well, gee, I don't know what to write [in the yearbook]. What did we do together this year?' And the other one said, 'Well, we got drunk a lot.' It's like if you got drunk or stoned together you are supposed to automatically become great friends and it just doesn't work that way. I think that's stupid, but I think that a lot of people believe it."

The second scenario called on the teenagers to compare situations that varied in the degree of risk involved:

I want you to think about two situations. In one, a group of friends decided to skip school and go to the beach at Jordan Lake. In the other, they went to the beach on a Saturday. Are the friends likely to feel closer in one situation or another, or not necessarily? Why? Now consider a third situation in which the friends went to a neighborhood barbecue with their families. How does this situation compare with the other two in terms of how the friends feel about each other? Why?

Responses to these scenarios were also remarkably consistent. In comparing the two beach situations, fully 90% of the teenagers claimed that skipping school, more than going on a Saturday, would be attended by feelings of interpersonal closeness. Three categories of reasons predominated. One stressed secrecy, privacy, and freedom (30%): "You have a secret that you share"; "No one else is around so you can do what you want." Another emphasized how the novelty of skipping school would create memories to share down the road (25%). Apropos of the argument regarding risk and narrative, one said, "They'd be closer if they skipped school because it's something new they've done together, and they'll all have to make up a story." The last category of responses referred to passing a test, surviving an ordeal, or proving one's commitment to the group (45%, most of whom were males): "You feel like you've made it through something together"; "You're rebellious together—you beat the establishment together"; "It shows what lengths you'll go to be with the group."

For the same reasons that skipping school was invested with greater symbolic significance and interpersonal meaning, attending a neighborhood barbecue was derided:

> "They would have a lot less fun [at the barbecue] because when you're with your friends you don't really have to conform to anything like your parents or your brothers or sisters, being careful to always be what they want. If you're comfortable with your friends then you can just be yourself. I usually have a lot more fun with just my friends because I can act more naturally."

In equal numbers (90%), and with equal vehemence, the teenagers argued that such an event would have no effect on the characters' relationships with one another. The most common reason provided referred to the absence of privacy or freedom (70%): "You have to act like your parents expect you to act so you can't be as free"; "Parents are gross and you can't talk seriously in front of them"; "It's not of your own will, your parents made you go." The remainder referred to the lack of shared excitement, sense of ordeal, or rebelliousness. There was unanimity among those in the 10% who believed, in contrast to the majority, that interpersonal inroads could be made at a barbecue. To wit, "they'd be united in thinking it was stupid."

Risks are extra-ordinary by these reports. They are a fount of memories and secrets, of shared knowledge and experience, and invested with the meanings of group identity. Shared risks are seen as instrumental in the development of interpersonal relationships and group cohesion, and are often described as symbolic or demonstrative of such relationships. Moreover, the meanings inscribed in risk activities are seen to vary according to the social-psychological histories of those involved: For those in the process of forging a collective identity, shared risks are understood to provide an interpersonal, experiential conduit for entering or forming a group; for those whose relational histories are more articulated and secure, risks take on meaning as icons of identity. In either case, the adolescent's relational history is of high relevance to what it means to take a risk, and risk involvement, in turn, is an expression of who one is and would like to become. It is prospectively oriented, largely experimental, and, in these respects, a hopeful sort of activity.

Bound as it is to processes of social positioning, identity is inherently contrastive. This is particularly apparent in the way that risks and adventures are composed into stories that make them intelligible as icons of social identity (Harré, 1975). Ethnographic analyses of hunting and fishing stories, and stories of war and other contacts with outsiders find that such narratives promote a sense of shared history and community by mediating ingroup–outgroup relations. These social dramas, like other texts, narratives, and novels, stress suspense and improvisation, challenge and imagination, by which participants experience themselves as main characters in their own stories (Rosaldo, 1986). Scheibe (1986) believes that adventures provide particularly potent material for building and maintaining life stories, and Gergen and Gergen (1983) make a similar point with their concept of *dramatic engagement*. They argue that precipitous events, either positive or negative, are necessary ingredients for continued emotional investment in a narrative. The adolescents interviewed were virtually unanimous in believing that today's risks are tomorrow's memories: "The friends you have right now are the best you'll ever have, so you do things with them so that you can remember."

CHAPTER 6

Risk-Taking and the Architecture of Adolescent Society

with Jean Louis Gariépy

> When shall we open our minds to the conviction that the
> ultimate reality of the world is neither matter nor spirit, is
> no definite thing, but a perspective?
> —José Ortega y Gasset

Some years ago I worked in a program for teenage mothers and their babies, most of whom were white and middle-class, or Hispanic and poor. One day a Hispanic mother was accused of stealing a cosmetic bag from the purse of a white mother. A vicious fight rapidly organized along racial lines, and in the course of a morning moved by fits and starts throughout the building: an incident in the bathroom, then the hallway, the smoking room, the math class. Meaning to quell emotions, and reestablish order and routine, the program director called all of the young women into a large meeting room and proceeded to ask questions about who was accused by whom, of what crime, on the basis of what evidence, and so forth. Her plan backfired. More insults were exchanged and another fist-

This chapter was written with the assistance of Jean Louis Gariépy, currently with the Faculty of Psychology at the University of North Carolina, Chapel Hill. Professor Gariépy was instrumental in devising the general logic of the statistical analyses.

fight seemed imminent. Just then Cecilia stood up and reminded everyone that their babies were all downstairs playing, eating, or sleeping together in the day care, and asked whether the common challenge in trying to get by as teen mothers didn't supersede ethnic differences—or at least mascara.

The change in the emotional tone that pervaded the room was remarkable. This is not to suggest that everyone became best buddies, or that things weren't tense for a while. But there were no more angry or violent outbursts. With sage-like clarity Cecilia conjured a point of view that was more compelling, more real, than the definitions they had of themselves as Hispanic or white, or as ripped off or falsely accused, or as whatever else permitted acts of violence of one against another. A perspective was introduced, a certain cultural narrative invoked, a "grammar of motives" (Burke, 1966) imposed, and the meanings of actions were fixed accordingly.

The example is meant to illustrate how individuals organize action and experience in light of who they understand themselves to be. Although Cecilia was able to summon a different frame of mind, it would be wrong to conclude that such perspectives change kaleidoscopically or capriciously. As both the source and the outcome of interpretive activity, they are hard-won, ontogenetic affairs. From the point of view developed here, they are social-psychological constructions that organize and give form to the media through which identities are expressed and come into contact with others: mind, as constituted in language, symbol, and ceremony.

This particular take on *frame of mind,* or *perspective* as a structuring of activity and meaning has much in common with classical theories of role taking (e.g., Mead, 1934), and reference groups (Sherif & Sherif, 1964; Sherif et al., 1961; Shibutani, 1955). Both of these theories, as discussed in Chapter 2, provide insight into the manner by which individuals become capable of participating in the symbolic practices of their social communities. Mead's role-taking theory, remember, suggests that persons distinguish themselves as members of a community to the degree that they permit the attitudes of others to enter into their own immediate expressions. In other terms, the height of social participation and cultural connectedness is also the height of self-development, and both take their measure from the extent to which persons "call out" in themselves the attitudes of others—the extent to which they take the role of other. Reference group theory, as articulated by Sherif and Shibutani, is cast in a comparable mold. To participate socially, in these terms, is to construct a frame of reference that organizes action and provides a psychological anchor for members of the community. Group norms, codes of conduct, and other symbols of social identity structure the actions and experiences of group members. The developmental argument concerns the way that perspectives are transformed in the course of coordinating one's own point of view with those of others. It is thus through members' participation in common communication channels that perspectives become shared and internalized as "a structure of expectations imputed to some audience for whom one organizes his conduct" (Shibutani, 1955, p. 565).

Coupled with the results presented in the previous chapter, these ideas make a case for a more direct examination of risks and peer group culture. How does risk-taking as social action also reflect perspective or point of view? How do they cohere? How does each explicate the other? Our theoretical confrontation with the connections between shared experience and the development of self and peer culture provides guidelines for understanding risk-taking as a type of text construction that expresses and generates personal and social identities. The relations between risks and peer culture will be explored in five groups of adolescents who present different patterns of risk involvement that cohere remarkably well with their more general social activity. However, addressing these issues empirically presents a difficult methodological task.

DEFINING PEER CULTURE

One of the most pressing concerns is that of defining and identifying the "peer group"—that carrier of the collective culture. It is clear from the developmental literature that investigators of children's social groups have been playing fast and loose with the term, referring variously to patterns of interaction manifested at a particular moment in time, or to a child's ongoing relationship with particular friends, or even the child's relationship with their entire generation. Inroads have been made to systematizing the language by distinguishing between, for example, group "structural" properties (e.g., relative size, or relative diversity in age and gender) and "relational" properties (e.g., cliquishness) (Ladd, 1983). However, it is difficult to address issues of group *culture* from this point of departure. Brown (1990) would like to resurrect some version of Dunphy's (1963) distinction between *cliques* and *crowds*, arguing that cliques are interaction-based associations whereas crowds are larger, reputation-based collectives from which individuals derive their cultural identities (jocks, nerds, druggies, etc.). In the case of the clique, norms are generated within the group; in the case of the crowd, they are imposed from without.

Efforts to introduce a more systematic taxonomy of groups represent an important conceptual step toward more dynamic and inclusive accounts of children's social lives. Still, the research strategies typically employed—traditional observational and sociometric techniques, for example—which may be adequate for tracking young children's peer relations, become inordinately cumbersome for following the complicated social lives of adolescents. But more than these practical matters, the concerns with group size, demography, the number of times that particular individuals are mentioned as belonging to a group (often used to index "popularity"), and so forth, carry the great danger of distraction, of turning us away from the customs, meanings, cultural practices, and shared experiences that psychologically anchor individuals to one another, and provide the material out of which they fashion a sense of "us." As Geertz (1983) has made plain, to adopt an interpretive approach is to shift modes of thought to those "rather more familiar to the translator, the exegete, or iconographer than to the test giver, the factor analyst, or the pollster" (p. 31).

Nevertheless, it is not my intention to debate the relative merits of qualitative versus quantitative analysis. My purpose is to identify the architecture—the structure, organization, or form—of adolescent social groups as it relates to the development and instantiation of shared symbolic activity. Both types of analysis are employed to this end. What needs to be emphasized, however, is that issues of analysis were initiated and resolved within a broader explanatory perspective in which social participation and culture are understood to be dialectially coordinated and peer groups are understood as open, interacting, and dynamic systems.

CROWD TYPES

We begin, first, with adolescents' perceptions of the larger social scene. Participants were asked to list and provide brief descriptions of the different crowd types (i.e., "Tell me about the different groups, the preppies, jocks, etc."). Eight such crowd types were named: punks, preps, rednecks, blacks, nerds, hippies, drammies, and norms. A variety of distinguishing features were discussed, including style of dress, shared activities, sport preferences, drug preferences, the sorts of cars that they drive—even where the cars are parked in the high school lot. Another mark of distinction was the Main Street hangout. A Friday or Saturday evening stroll down Main Street will confirm that it is a Mecca for area teenagers, who colonized various places according to whether they are punks or hippies or rednecks and so forth, according to their crowd type.

Punks, known also as *rebels* (especially among themselves), smoke cigarettes, wear black, and like to fight. They sport Mohawk hair styles. Typically, their ears are pierced extensively. They are known for their heavy drug use: pot, alcohol, cocaine, and LSD are all used frequently and in large quantities. There aren't many punks in the area, but they stand out, strategically, as weird. They drive weird cars, dress weird, and act weird: "I had one in my class and she felt under her desk and found some bubble gum and picked it off and started chewing it." On Friday and Saturday nights, punks can be found on Main Street, hanging out in front of a particular sandwich shop.

Preps, also referred to as *rich country clubbies*, or *socies*, are from upper-class families. "The boys are jocks; the girls are beautiful." They are confident. They play tennis and soccer, wear nice clothes, and get brand new cars for their 16th birthdays—"fancy ones, better than what my dad drives." Their parents are less restrictive, and they take more risks, these perhaps related. Preps smoke cigarettes, get drunk and stoned, and they have tried cocaine. One of the most salient group features was their cliquishness: "they're snobs"; "snobby"; "snobs, all of them." The exception is the *smart populars*, who do well in school, and are considerably less elitist. No Main Street hangout was mentioned.

Rednecks, or *hicks*, come from lower-class backgrounds. They are loud and mean and like to have fun. They drive cars fast, but not fast cars. They wear boots, denim, hats, and shades. They display Confederate flags on their cars or trucks, play football, like to fight. Alcohol and pot are the drugs of choice. They do poorly in school, and don't mind: "Not much stress is put on education by their parents." They park their cars in the "lower lot." Their Main Street hangout is in front of a video arcade.

Blacks, also called *homeboys* and *homegirls*, were described as spending time only with each other. This was more or less true of the other group descriptions as well; however, the relative lack of contact between blacks and the other groups was strongly evident in how infrequently they were mentioned by the predominantly white participants. The few individuals who described this group did so in terms similar to those used to described rednecks: Blacks are from lower-class backgrounds, mean (especially the girls), do poorly in school, and like to fight. Like the rednecks, they also hang out in front of the video arcade; most of the fights are between blacks and rednecks. Most blacks do not drive cars, presumably for reasons of an economic nature. In fact, one of only a few black teens interviewed distinguished between two black groups on the basis of economic status and aspirations. In both groups, however, there was a decided racial segregation: "Most of the time blacks and whites do not mix much. The blacks are divided into two groups, the kind who are lower class and not as goal oriented, and the middle-class blacks. I'm smart and have a lot of intellectual friends who are usually white, and I have a black friend. They don't really mix together, they [blacks and whites] don't usually get along, so I'm always the butterfly."

Nerds were described as "chumps," "losers," and "left-overs." They seem not to care about how they appear to others: "They don't spend much time making themselves look nice." Nerds are known for not taking risks, probably best expressed by the comment, "I never hear any stories about them." They do not party or have many friends. They take school seriously, staying in at lunch to do their homework, but many do not do very well. They are "ugly" and "act dumb," the latter because they are "socially inept." Indeed,

they are universally annoying in their "wannabe" manner of following others around. No Main Street hangout was mentioned.

Hippies, junior Woodstocks, or *heads* wear tie-dye, peace emblems,
and long hair. Considered a gentle group, they play music—folk and
early '60s rock and roll—and are "easy to talk to." Some described
them as politically savvy: "really into knowing stuff—current events
and stuff." Like punks, hippies are reputed to use drugs excessively,
especially pot and LSD. They hang out and play music on the front
steps of a large Main Street office building.

Drammies are those who participate in the school plays. They
park their cars in a lot adjacent to the theater building, where they
spend most of their free time. They are politically and socially liber-
al. Indeed, open-mindedness and acceptance of individual differences, or better, personal flair, is cultivated with a vengeance: "We
tend to look for people who are not shy or withdrawn, people who
can stand out and be funny, and that kind of thing. We accept people who are willing to take a chance socially. We usually talk to new
people and try to get to know them. Then usually they don't fit in
with us, and they go off." Others consider them clannish in the extreme.

Finally are the *norms, regulars,* or *moderates,* who come from mid-
dle- and upper-middle-class families. They wear jeans and tee shirts.
They are smart, good at sports, active, "have lots of ambitions."
Their parents are well educated, many holding faculty positions at
local universities. Some of their interests and activities connect
them, to some extent, with other crowd types: "They're sort of a
mix of the other types"; "I like redneckish stuff like hunting and
four-wheel driving, but also preppish stuff like going to parties while
parents are out of the country, and driving around in Dad's sports
car. But basically, I'm normal"; "I'm in between a punk and a
prep"; "I'm between a prep and a nerd."

The difficulty in stereotyping this particular group is expressed
by the following:

"The people that I hang out with are in the normal group, but
one of the preps would probably call us nerds. I'm sure all of
them would look down on us because we are not that distinct.
It's stupid. We would just be kind of there. A popular snob
would classify our group as nerds, but a popular smart would

not classify us. I wouldn't become close friends with a snob. Out of the groups, I would probably be friends with the drammies or the popular smart people."

Perhaps this group's membership is more variable than the others, as suggested above. On the other hand, the sampling method was such that most of the teenagers interviewed belonged to the "normal" group, and it may be, as one particularly insightful teenager declared, that "from the inside all groups are more diverse than from the outside." Indeed, several individuals refused to attach a crowd label to themselves until they were asked how they might be perceived by others. One, made up in black leather, black hair dye, black nail polish, and raccoon-mask makeup, insisted, "I'm just myself," but responded without hesitation to a prompt regarding the opinions of others: "Definitely punk." Said another, "I don't know what I am, but someone who's not my friend would probably say I'm a snob." The degree to which these crowd types are stereotyped, reputation based, and nearly institutionalized is further suggested by the adolescent who commented, "Well, I'm in the school plays, but I'm not a drammie person."

With the exception of nerds and rednecks, all of the crowd types described above were represented in the sample of individuals who were interviewed. We turn now to the methodological issues that frame the next portion of the study. The principal concern is how to conceptualize the connections between shared risks and social integration. We shall see that these connections are made at two levels. One level connects individuals to others within their immediate peer group; the other level connects specific peer groups to the larger community of teens, to adolescent society.

A METHODOLOGICAL FRAME

In order to guard and examine the connections between shared risk experience and peer culture, "peer groups" were defined and statistically identified on the basis of collective risk involvement; on the basis, that is, of each subject's nominations of individuals with whom they share risk experiences.

The process of identifying groups of risk-takers was facilitated by the cluster sampling method used for recruiting. Recall that it began with a personal contact who was asked for names of others who might be interested in participating. If they were willing, these individuals were interviewed and also asked for names of potential subjects. Thus, all of the teenagers were more or less closely associated with one another, which accounts for the homogeneity of the sample (predominantly white, middle-class high school students), as well as the occasional exception (Asians, blacks, high school dropouts, Quaker Friends School students).

The statistical procedures that were employed to determine the membership composition of the groups have proven useful for describing the social networks of other populations (e.g., aggressive children, Cairns et al., 1988; and school dropouts, Cairns, Cairns, & Neckerman, 1989). Briefly, they provided information about each individual's association with all other subjects in the sample, that is, each subject's *social profile*. Groups were then identified on the basis of similarities observed among social profiles. For example, if three individuals all nominated only one another as partners in risk, and were not so named by anyone else in the sample, they would have highly similar (in fact, perfectly correlated) social profiles, and would comprise an unambiguous group. Clearly, this textbook example of a perfectly reciprocated (every member names all other members) and self-contained group is just that. Intuitively, and as will be shown for the present sample, it is unlikely that each and every group member will nominate all other members, that is, show perfect reciprocity; it is also unlikely that all group members will show absolutely no association with individuals from other groups.

This state of affairs illustrates two additional features of group relations (beyond membership composition) that were tapped by the statistical procedures and that will be shown to have the utmost relevance for understanding the relationship between risk involvement and social participation: the degree of intragroup *cohesion*, and the extent of intergroup contact, or *permeability*. Cohesion was indexed by the average correlation of social profiles of individuals identified as belonging to the same group. This measure evaluates the relative strength or "tightness" of relationships within a particular collective. Permeability, on the other hand, refers to outside-group associations, or what might also be called intergroup contact. It reflects the degree to which specific groups are nested within, or isolated from, a broader and more inclusive system of social relationships. Using Dunphy's (1963) language, cohesion measures the interpersonal closeness of the clique, whereas permeability measures the clique's integration with the crowd.

Having established a strategy for identifying social groups within the sample, we may turn our hand to the task of examining the relationships between specific risk behaviors and peer group life. If risk activities are social commentaries that interpret the social-cognitive realities of those who enact and share them, we can expect within-group consensus regarding types of behaviors that members report as "risky." That is, group members should share a point of view from which to evaluate the meaning of behaviors as "risky." Moreover, beyond reconstructing the interpersonal dynamic that operates *within* groups, risk activities may also be expected to reflect dynamics operating *between* groups. For example, in a community of teens for which drinking alcohol and smoking pot are considered "normative" in the sense of being relatively common and socially acceptable, and carrying a weapon is considered "marginal," those who engage in the former should participate more fully in the larger community of teens, whereas those who participate in the latter should be more isolated from that community. In other words, more intergroup contact is expected in the first case, and more social isolation in the second. Thus, the marginality of risks should cohere with the marginality of groups.

This implication finds some support in the form of a study conducted by Cairns and his colleagues (Cairns et al., 1988), who studied the role of peer groups in fostering and maintaining deviant behavior. They found that although highly aggressive adolescents form social groups that are organizationally comparable to nonaggressive groups (also see Hubba et al., 1979), they are unpopular in the social network at large. It was speculated that individuals within aggressive cliques may be more likely to drop out of school due to rejection or expulsion, and have difficulty becoming integrated into the larger community. Additional evidence for the relative social isolation of groups engaged in marginal risk behaviors comes from a study of high school and college students' perceptions of common crowd types (e.g., brains, jocks, druggies, populars, toughs; Brown et al., 1990). Students reported that druggies and toughs were more likely to be socially disruptive, to hang out in out of the way places, and were less likely to be involved in extracurricular activities, compared to individuals in less deviant crowds.

All of this provides at least some tentative form of support for the argument that risk activities are social practices that reconstruct a history of peer group relations. They also make a strong case for moving beyond characterizations of peer groups as self-contained social units that operate in isolation from other social systems. Understanding adolescents' risks as social action requires a sensitivity not only to the structure of associations within particular peer groups, but between groups, or within a larger social network—a sensitivity, that is, to both intra- and intergroup relations, to the architecture of social groups.

DETERMINING GROUP MEMBERSHIP

The first analytic task was to identify discrete social groups within the sample. This was accomplished by examining individuals' nominations of their partners in risk (i.e., "Most people have a group of friends that they're more likely to do risky and adventurous things with; who's in your group?"). The original pool of 41 adolescents was reduced to 36 because 5 individuals did not nominate, nor were they nominated by anyone else in the sample as partners in risk, presumably because members of their particular peer groups were not interviewed. Responses from the remaining participants were organized into a 36 × 36 co-occurrence matrix. This involved tallying the number of times, across individuals, that any two were named together to the same group, that is, the number of times two individuals "co-occur" (these frequencies were entered as off-diagonal elements), and the number of times each individual was named to any group (entered as diagonal elements).

Table 6.1 is based on bogus data, but illustrates the procedures involved in constructing a co-occurrence matrix.

In this example, David (Dav) reported that he did risky and adventurous things with Andy (And) and Steve (Ste), so all three received a count on their respective diagonals for being mentioned at all, and all pair-wise possibilities received a count on the appropriate off-diagonals (i.e., Dav/And, Dav/Ste, And/Ste). Applied to the six respondents in this hypothetical sample, the resulting symmetrical

TABLE 6.1. Example of a Co-Occurrence Matrix

	And	Dav	Ste	Mar	Sta	Isa
And	3	3	3	—	—	—
Dav	3	3	3	—	—	—
Ste	3	3	3	1	—	—
Mar	—	—	1	4	2	2
Sta	—	—	—	2	2	1
Isa	—	—	—	2	1	2

matrix preserves each individual's (column) relationship with all other individuals (rows) in the sample, and thus provides a descriptive account of each person's "social profile." From here, it is possible to obtain estimates of similarities between individual profiles by inter-correlating the columns of the matrix. So the column that describes David's co-occurrence with all other individuals would be correlated with the column that describes Andy's co-occurrence with all other individuals, and so forth. The result is a symmetrical matrix of correlations. (Obviously, Andy, David, and Steve are perfectly correlated with each other, whereas the other subjects are not.)

The next step is to identify distinct clusters of individuals whose profiles are highly correlated with each other. The bogus co-occurrence matrix suggests two distinct clusters, marginally joined by an association between Steve and Mary (Mar). A statistical analysis of a more complicated data set can be accomplished in several ways (Gower, 1987; Green, 1989), two of which were used here— hierarchical cluster analysis and principal coordinate analysis (Legendre, 1976). The literature on clustering and ordination techniques recommends that cluster solutions be validated against the results of an ordination technique (Legendre, 1976; Sneath & Sokal, 1973). Both analytic techniques produce indices of similarities (or proximities) of individual profiles from the correlation matrix described above. However, in the case of hierarchical cluster analysis, the indices are correlations (i.e., individual profile correlations within the matrix are standardized), whereas in the case of principal coordinate analysis, the indices are Euclidean distances between individual profile correlations.

The initial hierarchical cluster analysis indicated that six individuals (all girls) formed dyads that were not associated with other individuals in the sample. The data that they provided were not included in subsequent analyses so as to maximize within-cluster similarities and between-cluster differences. In other words, including their data would have diluted the strength of correlations within and between groups, making group boundaries less discernible. Discarding data from three dyads of girls raises some concern regarding gender differences in social relationships, and introduces the possibility of gender bias in the remaining pool of respondents. That is, it might be the case that adolescent girls are likely to hang out in pairs, whereas boys are more likely to hang out in groups. In this case, however, the "pairs" were an artifact resulting from not interviewing the remaining members of the girls' peer groups. It should be noted as well that material provided by one boy was excluded, because he changed groups midway through the data collection phase.

New co-occurrence and correlation matrices were generated for the 29 individuals remaining. The hierarchical cluster analysis was repeated for the reduced matrix, generating the dendrogram shown in Figure 6.1 where five discrete clusters may be discerned. The five groups differed in size and sex ratio, as indicated by the code running down the left of the figure. Groups 1 and 2 consisted of six and four males, respectively. The other three groups were of mixed gender: Group 3 included two females (one Asian) and one male; Group 4 included six females (one black) and two males; Group 5 included seven males (one shcool dropout, one parochial school student) and one female (a school dropout). Note that this last group contained a peripheral member only marginally associated with the other individuals. Group 4 also included a likely peripheral member, although her relative association to the group was stonger than that of the peripheral male in Group 5, owing to the lesser strength of association of her group as a whole.

Results from the hierarchical clustering procedure were validated against a principal coordinate analysis, which generated comparable information regarding the constitution of the five groups.

GROUP STRUCTURAL PROPERTIES

In addition to generating information about the content of social clusters (i.e., the specific individuals belonging to each group), the

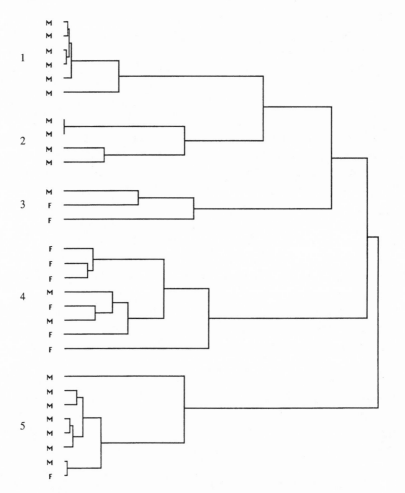

FIGURE 6.1. Hierarchical cluster analysis of social groups.

two analyses present consistent information about the structural features of specific groups. The first property concerns relative *cohesion*. As shown in the dendrogram of Figure 6.1, individuals in Groups 1 and 5 clustered at higher correlational levels compared to individuals in the other three groups. To obtain a more explicit estimate of group cohesion, the individual profile correlations within each group were examined.

Table 6.2 shows individual profile correlations within each

TABLE 6.2. Individual Profile Correlations within Groups

Group 1

	1	2	3	4	5	6
1	—	.98	.97	.77	.98	.93
2		—	.99	.80	.99	.96
3			—	.78	.99	.98
4				—	.80	.79
5					—	.96
6						—

Group 2

	1	2	3	4
1	—	1.0	.58	.53
2		—	.58	.53
3			—	.86
4				—

Group 3

	1	2	3
1	—	.71	.56
2		—	.46
3			—

Group 4

	1	2	3	4	5	6	7	8
1	—	.76	.93	.90	.76	.76	.65	.44
2		—	.66	.65	.84	.84	.68	.20
3			—	.95	.63	.63	.53	.74
4				—	.54	.54	.45	.66
5					—	.90	.82	.16
6						—	.82	.16
7							—	.12
8								—

Group 5

	1	2	3	4	5	6	7	8
1	—	.95	.94	.98	.93	.94	.90	.55
2		—	.88	.95	.84	.85	.95	.51
3			—	.97	.85	.84	.89	.64
4				—	.85	.86	.93	.63
5					—	.99	.77	.39
6						—	.77	.38
7							—	.70
8								—

cluster. Here it can be seen that the correlations for Groups 1 and 5 were high relative to the other three groups, with the exception of the peripheral member of Group 5. Interestingly, this particular individual lived some miles out of town, and his participation in group activities, especially on evenings and weekends, was curtailed by transportation difficulties. His low correlations within the group reflect the fact that his nominations were generally not reciprocated, and I suspect that his irregular involvement in collective risk-taking accounts for this.

The mean of individual profile correlations within each group was adopted as an index of group cohesion. The means for Groups 1 through 5 were .91, .68, .58, .76, and .90 respectively, indicating that Groups 1 and 5 are indeed more cohesive relative to the other three (the mean correlation for Group 5 was calculated without the peripheral member).

The second group structural feature concerns the *permeability* of group boundaries, or the extent to which members have contact, risk-wise, with individuals from outside their immediate social cluster. This measure of intergroup relations is intended to cast light on the degree to which groups are integrated within the larger teen community. This was explored by examining nominations, made or received, involving nongroup individuals, and comparing those frequencies to what would be expected by chance (i.e., under the assumption that the nominations would be randomly distributed within the network).

Figure 6.2 shows the deviations from expected values for both *nominations of* nongroup members and *nominations by* nongroup members. Three markedly different patterns of permeability are apparent. Group 1 stands apart as being more "attractive" than the others, and not at all inclined to nominate outsiders. By contrast, individuals of Group 4, and especially Group 5, tended neither to nominate nor to be nominated by outsiders. In fact, members of these two groups were *never* nominated by outsiders as partners in risk. It is worth noting, however, that nominations of outsiders were distributed across 3 individuals in Group 4, and produced by only one individual in Group 5—the peripheral member. Groups 2 and 3 constitute a third unique pattern in that their attractiveness and their interest in outsiders show little deviation from expected values.

Based on these analyses, Group 5 stands apart from the others

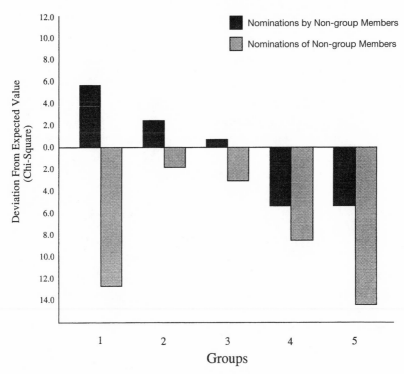

FIGURE 6.2. Deviations from expected values for outside-group nominations.

in the extent of its social isolation. Its singularity in this respect was apparent in several other areas as well. When asked for names of individuals that they hung out with now and again, but not on a regular basis, the members of other groups provided large lists whereas members of Group 5 provided absolutely none. Likewise, when polled informally about their plans for the future, members of other groups generated a variety of interests, all of which involved moving into new social circles. Those of Group 5, in contrast, wanted to stay together and become rock and roll stars.

At this point we have identified two structural features of adolescent social life—cohesion and permeability—which appear to be independent of one another. That is, group solidarity or cohesion, as measured by overlapping social profiles, is not necessarily isomorphic with the degree to which the system is open to external social influences. Nonetheless, these two dynamics may contribute simultaneously to individual social life and development: Whereas cohesion without permeability forecloses opportunities for new identifications, permeability in the absence of cohesion diffuses the social identifications presumed necessary for an enduring sense of selfhood. Social systems that foster solidarity within the collective, as well as interaction without, would appear to nourish the ongoing social-cognitive development of group members. In groups marked by a high degree of intragroup similarity or cohesion, and a low degree of permeability to external social forces, however, we can expect these dynamics to be diminished correspondingly.

SHARED RISKS AND PEER CULTURE

Having determined the content of particular peer groups, and having explicated differences in the structural properties of cohesion and permeability, the next task was to determine the extent to which the structure of particular groups cohered with the structure of risks reported by group members.

Table 6.3 catalogues the categories of risks reported across the five groups, and presents the proportion of individuals within each group who claimed to have experienced them.

These data were culled from two sources. One was a general question about the types of risky and adventurous things that group members do together; the other was a request for a personal story about a recent risk or adventure.

The procedures for clustering risks were similar to those described for clustering friends. That is, they began with the construction of co-occurrence and correlation matrices on the basis of risks reported by each individual in the sample. The dendrogram shown in Figure 6.3 illustrates results from the hierarchical clustering analysis.

The analysis suggests two primary clusters of risks, which were confirmed with a principal coordinate analysis. Those in the top group are generally regarded as mildly mischievous and "normative." Those in the bottom cluster, however, are legally and culturally sanctioned as "deviant," entail potential for more severe punishment, and are seen among a smaller proportion of adolescents.

TABLE 6.3. Categories of Risks Reported across Groups

Risk category	Group				
	1	2	3	4	5
Sneak out of house	50	25	50	57	50
Hang out uptown	67	0	0	43	17
Drive around looking for fun/parties	67	25	0	13	0
Drive fast/risky	67	50	33	25	14
Party	67	75	100	86	50
Drink alcohol	33	75	100	86	50
Drink alcohol	33	75	0	57	67
Pranks	0	0	0	29	67
Sneak into adult bars/ fraternity parties	0	0	0	29	67
Smoke marijuana	17	0	0	14	67
Fighting (at frat parties)	0	0	0	0	33
LSD (hallucinogenic drug)	0	0	0	0	43

It is noteworthy that the two classes of risk activity identified here (including the "dual membership" of drinking; i.e., it is common to both clusters of risks) reconstruct the cultural distinction generally made between "normative" and "deviant" forms of adolescent risk involvement. It is also essential to keep in mind that these classes could not have been distinguished if individuals had reported involvement in both of them. In other words, the teenagers were reporting involvement in either the normative type or the deviant type, but not both. Thus, while individuals tended to engage in more than one category of risk (e.g., drinking, sneaking out), they rarely engaged in more than one class of risk (normative or deviant). This bodes well for the theoretical expectation regarding the relationship between the marginality of risks, and the marginality of social groups. We are now well placed to consider whether members of the socially isolated group are those most involved in the deviant class of risk.

The analysis linking individuals' patterns of risk involvement with group membership involved calculating the percentages of individuals within each group who claimed to have experienced risks belonging to the two classes—normative and deviant. Not surprisingly, and as shown in Figure 6.4, all groups reported normative

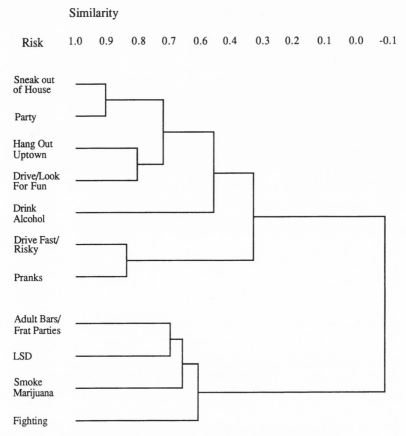

FIGURE 6.3. Hierarchical cluster analysis of risks.

kinds of risks, some more exclusively than others. Three patterns are discernible. One is associated with Groups 1 and 4, and characterized by a high degree of normative risks, and relatively few that belong to the deviant class. The second pattern, expressed by Groups 2 and 3, is characterized by less risk-taking generally, and a complete absence of the deviant categories. Finally, Group 5 exhibited a level of normative risk involvement similar to that of Groups 2 and 3, but distinguished itself from all groups by its marked propensity for deviant involvement.

Taken together, the results show a certain coherence between

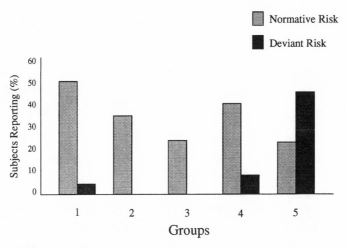

FIGURE 6.4. Percentages of subjects reporting normative and deviant risks.

the marginality of risk participation and the marginality of social groups. Group 5, the only one chararacterized by a major involvement in deviant activities, was also the only group to demonstrate both a high degree of internal cohesion as well as a low degree of permeability to the larger social network. While this group stands apart on the basis of the deviant risks reported, it is also interesting to consider the types of risks that are *not* reported. Specifically, members of this group are not particularly involved in the more normative forms (of 23 risks reported, only 7 were normative). They tend not to party, to drive around looking for parties, or to hang out uptown, all of which may be considered vehicles of social contact with the larger teen community.

Group 1 presents a different picture. It was the most active with respect to normative risk-taking, was as cohesive as Group 5, but considerably more popular in the larger network. This pattern fits that of popular individuals and leaders, who have been shown in sociometric studies to nominate each other preferentially (hence their high index of cohesion), and to receive more positive nominations compared to individuals classified as "average," "rejected," or "neglected" (see Kupersmidt & Patterson, 1991). Thus, in this case as well, risk involvement reconstructs the social history of the group.

SOCIAL PRACTICE AND CULTURAL MEANING

The manner by which collective risk-taking counts as both interpersonal activity and social commentary was apparent in the comparative analysis of the five groups, and showed that Group 5 displayed a unique pattern of social isolation with regard to both intergroup contact and the more private nature of its risk involvement. Interestingly, the extent of this isolation was very much apparent to the group members. In discussing the different social groups within the high school, for example, one individual ran through the laundry list of "punks," "rednecks," "nerds," "jocks," "norms," and then added the "outcasts," saying:

> "I guess that's what you'd call us. Each one of my close friends is extremely talented in some way: instrumentally, or singing, or dancing. We're all kind of outcasts and looked on as kind of weird. Every close friend of mine that I've ever known has either been a radical music lover or a very talented musician. We draw together. ["In what way are you outcasts?"] You don't go to school to learn anything about music or dancing; you have to go to a specialized school for that. The normal thing is menial work jobs or executive jobs, and the way musicians are looked on—we don't seem to fit into school."

In another discussion of how their group is perceived by outsiders, a different individual said that they were referred to as the "dirt-heads," because "they say we don't take baths, or change clothes, and our hair is dirty." Moments later, this individual described all group members as "extremely physically attractive." By both accounts, there is a marked discrepancy between their own perceptions, and their beliefs about the perceptions of other teenagers. They appear untouched by these potential conflicts, however, and unable to entertain the possible legitimacy of an alternative point of view. In this regard, their social isolation and their psychological disconnectedness may be understood as mutually constituting. They "don't seem to fit," nor have they constructed a frame of reference that extends beyond the group, and from which they might evaluate themselves. Stated somewhat differently, they recognize the authority of no perspective other than the one that gives meaning to the immediate and local goals and desires of themselves and their companions. Again, on the issue of social groups within the high school:

> "We try not to get into that [group affiliation] anymore, because they're all typical high school students. They'll go to college and they fit in with school. A lot of the people I hang out with are dropouts and we are extremely prejudiced against the great percentage of the school and we try not to get into that kind of grouping."

Said another, "I dropped out last March because I don't need school for what I want to do. I want to be a rock-and-roll star."

By choice, ostracism, or some combination of these, members of Group 5 were clearly disengaged from the teen community, and the extent of this isolation was instantiated in the privacy of risk-taking activities: "We used to go to parties where parents weren't there, and hang out and stuff, but now we know older people. Now we go to people who live by themselves." The primary activity at these social gatherings was taking drugs and listening to music.

PEER CULTURE AS PERSPECTIVE

Adolescent risk involvement and social life are not independent entities that can be placed in some mechanical, cause–effect relationship, no matter the elegance or complexity of the factorial design or path model within which that relationship is expressed. Particular risk forms do not cause social isolation; they manifest it. And when we acknowledge that action and meaning are internally related, when we connect "action to its sense rather than behavior to its determinants" (Geertz, 1983, p. 84), we take up the task of exploring how they are jointly composed—the task, that is, of interpretive explanation.

Such explanation is concerned to tell how actions are constructed and derive their meaning from a history of actions and shared experience, and how meaning is reconstituted in the process. We have here a hermeneutic circle—or spiral, as Dilthey prefers, because each turn transcends its predecessor. We have here, as well, the realization that what is created and recreated over time is a certain perspective. Modern adolescent society is a case in point:

In contemporary society, adolescents come into contact with a variety of groups that maintain a variety of perspectives. It seems likely, indeed necessary, that the criteria for inclusion, esteem, or stature—that definitions of identity—within children's groups have been recast from those that were once relevant. That is, in the mixed-age groups of years past, the strength and clarity of one's voice was probably granted according to one's years, and the experience and knowledge that cleave to them. But refracted through the many faces of modern mass society, children's social groups have become increasingly differentiated and spectral. Today's peer group *types* include punks, rednecks, preppies, druggies, nerds, dead heads, tree-huggers, and norms, to name just a few, and this diversity indicates the extent to which contemporary adolescents must sort themselves out along new and different dimensions, and take a more deliberate part in establishing and maintaining their place in the social scheme of things (the part in this process played by risk-taking, as cultural experience, is clear). The transformation is clearly sociocultural in that it creates new roles, voices, and names to adopt, speak, and address—new identity opportunities; but it is also epistemic, creating a higher order understanding, a greater reflective awareness of self in relation to others. Recent changes in the composition and structure of children's groups encourage a more conscious attention to the fact that one has friends, that friends form groups, that groups stand in relation to other groups. Thus, participating in the diversity and "polyphony" of modern life provides more than a sea of alternatives for one's social identity; it contributes to the awareness that one *has* a social identity.

Sociocultural and epistemic processes—identity and reflective awareness—move forward in tandem as *perspective*. Indeed, if interpretive activity could be said to have a purpose, it would be the clarity of perspective (Lightfoot, in press-a). This conclusion may be seen to repose on the cognitive developmental position that the peer group is a primary source of novelty and conflict which moves individuals along a path toward increasing decentration (e.g., Inhelder & Piaget, 1958; Piaget, 1965/1995; Selman, 1980; Youniss & Smollar, 1985). It is the "pressure of contact with other minds and other viewpoints" (Chapman, 1991, p. 220) that provokes a more objective stance toward self and others.

This position is presaged by a history of social cognitive research that points to the vital connections between peer relations and self-reflection. Recall from Chapter 2 Inhelder and Piaget's (1958) thesis that peer group activities promote decentration and the ability to reflect on and mediate one's own actions on the basis of perceived ideas, ideals, and ideologies of a wider group. Several research programs have been devoted to pursuing this thesis. Selman (1980), for example, reasoned that peer social interactions provide a source of "conceptual conflict" between one's own ideas and those of others. Exposure to different ideas, perspectives, modes of reasoning, and so forth are understood to provoke conflict and promote a greater depth of understanding of oneself and the social systems in which one participates. Similarly, Youniss and Smollar (1985) argued that social participation and relationships are fundamental and not simply derivative characteristics of intrapersonal selfhood:

> In the view we are proposing, the self relies on relationships and needs them to escape egoism. Self-understanding does not proceed solely through private discourse wherein the self reflects on its own reasoning. That leads to an internal spiral of infinite regression in which a self could become embedded in its own subjectivity. The way out of this inward tunnel is to take one's reflections to others for their review. It is through the movement outward that the self can learn whether others understand it and find out how others have reasoned about similar topics. (p. 169)

For Youniss and Smollar, adolescent friendships serve important developmental functions. They argued, in fact, that relations with others constitute "correctives" against exaggerated feelings of uniqueness (1985, p. 138). It is in the context of sharing concerns, solving problems, forming ideas and opinions—in essence, constructing intersubjective realities through participating in the communicative and symbolic practices of the peer group—that reflective awareness and social identification take place.

CHAPTER 7

Pursuing Depth

There hangs about all our knowledge, in fact, a
future-ward reference, as actual in our meaning as
the post-ward.

—JAMES MARK BALDWIN

It happens typically that when we look for contributions to current
behavior and experience, we reach into the past. It may be an ancient and unremembered past—some evolutionary species adaptation, perhaps, or cultural template, or archaic consciousness. On a
different scale, it may be a past defined by the life history of the individual—one that harbors a singular, formative event, or one that
contains a collection of events, or a repetitious pattern of experience that culminates over time until some epigenetic threshold of
significance is breached. The past may also be that of only a moment ago, something just said, or felt, or understood.

Coursing through all of these possibilities is a tendency to regard current actions as outcomes that are preceded in time by particular causes, a tendency that flows staunchly and unimpeded
within traditional psychological research. However, cultural experience—risk-taking, play, science, art—will not submit to this interpretation, and puts to rout our habit of viewing experience as the
present effects of things past. To neglect the way that actions are
mobilized in pursuit of a partially unknown, though nevertheless
real and tangible future is to dismantle the epistemological scaffold
of the organismic tradition—the constructive, semiotically mediated, and temporally organized nature of human development. It is
to deny the future-ward reference that hangs about all our knowledge.

In this book I have tried to set forth a developmental and thus dynamic account of adolescent risk-taking. However, whereas all developments are by definition dynamic, not everything dynamic constitutes development; and because there has arisen a confusion on this point in recent years, I have devoted considerable effort to elaborating a theoretical perspective from which to bring the developmental and future-ward relevance of risk-taking into focus. In the pages to follow I would like to enunciate certain points of this perspective, and draw out a few theoretical and practical implications. My intention is that they be read as a condensation of an organismic narrative in which child development is understood to be "a temporal operation par excellence."

THE INTENT TO BE A SUBJECT

Much of the argument set forth in preceeding chapters turns on the assumption that adolescent risk-taking is not a *behavior* so much as it is a manifestation of a basic social-psychological process. This process shows itself most visibly and vividly in what we typically label "play" when it occurs in younger children, and "science" or "art" in the case of adults. The underlying process is therefore not limited to adolescence, but is a fundamental feature of all knowledge construction. In his *Meditations on Quixote*, Ortega y Gasset (1914/1961) expresses exactly this point when he writes that the very structure of life is a way of being what one still is not. To root oneself in trying, seeking, and desiring; to define one self and be judged on the basis of acts of *will*; to apprehend reality by embracing the unforeseen, the un-thought-of, and the new—this is what it means to be a hero, to be capable of *taking* a risk and *having* experience.

This is all very much in line with Baldwin's description of *the intent to be a subject* (1908). He couples this to his idea of the future-oriented nature of all knowledge, and implicates the forward pressing and accommodative activity of self as instrumental in its own further development. At issue, in particular, is the development of self-reflection and all that it entails, most notably the experience of self as a singular center of inner processes, and the identification with others whose inwardness and subjectivity is similarly recognized and appreciated. The intent to be a subject is thus bound up with the constitution of the object-self, that is, the objective, empirical self that one thinks about, is embarrassed by, makes excuses for, and justifies to oneself and others. The object-self leans into the future as hypothesis, as exteriorizations of desire and yearning, as the imagination of something that may become truth. It pulls forward in its wake its own interlocutor, the subject-self; the known, actual, taken for granted, and true self. And it is a genuine interlocutor, not something after the fact caught in the dynamic whorl of imagination in action. The subject-self provides the structure through which the object-self may be realized. In Baldwin's terms, the forward pressing, accommodative, and active life is mediated through a system of established ideas: "fulfillments of the external are prophesied" (1908, p. 413).

The empirical, objective, and imaginative, and the rational, subjective, and inferential: these are the two forms of self that take shape in the process of trying to be someone. Together they comprise a dialectical unity through which subject and object are jointly organized. Baldwin (1908) describes the process as one of "progressive determination" (p. 408), and his term is as good as any for capturing some notion of the dynamic structure, or structured dynamic, or what Valsiner (1987) calls the "bounded indeterminancy" that constitutes the nature of development.

The seeds of Vygotsky's (1971) concern with this issue were sown early on. In his work on artistic creation, which predates his interest in developmental psychology, he distinguishes between the structural aspect of a composition—(in music, a melody; in literature, a narrative) and the dynamic aspect (its intention, purpose, and meaning). Structure and dynamic are unified in the constructive process. The dynamic aspect is crystallized, objectified, and embodied in the structure of the composition in much the same way that a physiological process inhabits the anatomical structure of an organ (Leontiev, 1971, p. viii). Or consider Ortega's metaphor of the stone: When thrown it carries within it the curve of its own flight. It is impulse embodied, which is to say, expressed, developed, and fulfilled. The form, the curve, contains the impulse that propels it, but presents it in a clear, articulated, and developed way (1914/1961, pp. 112–113).

It becomes especially apparent in light of earlier discussions of his work that Baldwin understands the progressive organization of self to be but an example of the more general development of knowledge and consciousness. The constitution of the subject-self and the object-self reflect ongoing cycles between the known and the unknown, cycles (or spirals) that we have come to recognize as interpretive activity. This is an ever-present universal in the development of knowledge that applies equally to infant reflex and scientific hypothesis, as Overton (1994) points out. But although interpretive activity is not limited to conscious thought and reflection, I have argued here that thought becomes conscious and reflective because of it.

Like the child's play that precedes it, and the adult's creative work that follows, adolescent risk-taking expresses an intent to be a subject. In it we see a self forward pressing and hypothetical, but nevertheless structured and organized. It gestures toward the new, toward novelty and experience, but not just any experience is relevant; risk-taking is not an unbridled romp through the unknown. As Baldwin was at pains to point out, the noisy clash will lose interest whether in play or art. Risk, drama, play, cultural experience are all defined and derive their social-cognitive significance from the manner in which they are framed. This is experience organized as an intent to be a subject; it is art for the sake of self.

TROLL AND MAN

I recognize some need for clarification on this last issue—art for the sake of self—which follows Vygotsky's thesis on adolescent imagination and fantasy. The conception of self presented here has been at least partially eclipsed by an altogether new and different version: self as context. This immersion, or fusion, of persons and situations is generally accomplished in the name of *contextualism*, a local translation of the larger cultural movement of postmodernism (Chandler, 1993). By definition, and in contradistinction to modernism's metanarratives—its dialectical syntheses, hermeneutical meanings, emancipatory interests, and so forth—postmodernism "loses . . . its great hero, its great dangers, its great voyagers, its great goal" (Lyotard, 1984, p. xxiv). In this topsy-turvy world in which texts write authors, languages speak speakers, objects possess owners, and crimes commit themselves (Shalin, 1993, pp. 314–315), the self as individuated, agentic, continuous, and enduring has been fully censured. It has been judged a tyrant that by some accident of history rose to power and position to insist on its own authority, its own continuity and worth. Worse, it has been judged a ruse that creates a confusion between substance and appearance until an act of deconstruction expels the voices, texts, and codes that it conveys, leaving an empty integument behind. By this logic, and in Lyotard's words, "a *self* does not amount to much" (1984, p. 15; original italitcs).

The postmodernism that has so thoroughly engulfed contemporary thinking has been whipped to a froth by forces that are largely political. Believing the activity, agency, and transcendent authority of the "modern" self to be synonomous with oppression and a Nietzschean "will to power," postmodernism attenuates the self across a vast network of family, social, and cultural institutions in order to grant each voice equal weight regardless of race, class, or gender. The suspension of the usual social roles and ranks of individuals suggests an intent to reinstate something comparable to the Greek *polis*, a political system that assumed equality between all participants. As Tiresias shouted to Oedipus: "King though you are, one right—to answer—makes us equal!" Aristotle distinguished the *polis* from *societas*, a mere association of individuals brought together for a specific purpose—production, economic gain, and so forth—for which an unequal distribution of power or authority might be advantageous, and even necessary.

But such attentuation of self may undercut the very agenda set forth by postmodern activists, if granting authority to all, in the end, is the same as granting it to none. In other words, postmodernism incurs the great danger of creating a self so thinly spread that it lacks the depth of experience and understanding necessary to social commitment and moral conviction. We have, in this case, a self in the manner of Ibsen's Troll King, who puts to Peer Gynt the question, "What is the difference between Troll and Man?" and then, unhappy with Peer's reply, exclaims:

> I'll tell you what it is.
> Out there, under the shining vault of heaven,
> Men tell each other: "Man, be thyself!"
> But here, among us trolls, we say:
> "Troll, be thyself—*and thyself alone*. . . ."

"Thyself alone" distinguishes the Troll (see May, 1991). It is

> . . . never to care
> For the world beyond our frontier.

But for the man: These words—Be thyself!—carry the ancient wisdom of Polonius as he sends Laertes off to Paris:

> This above all: to thine own self be true
> And it doth follow, as the night the day,
> Thou canst not then be false to any man.

For Polonius, in contrast to the Troll King, being true to oneself is enobled by a larger purpose both moral and public. Being true to oneself is not an end, but a means of not being false to others (Trilling, 1971), and in this regard Polonius raises being a self to a higher plane. In uttering these immortal words, in fact, Polonius steps above his own small-minded, ineffectual, used up old man of a self, and adjures us to be something more heroic. This self is an obstinacy that refuses to yield to local taste and sentiment. It insists on itself! Leaving behind the path of convention for one that is more principled, it is someone for the sake of another. Throughout the long haul of history we have held fast to "This above all: to thine own self be true"; but recently, shorn of its predicate of not being false to others, the purpose is diminished. We have similarly obscured the purpose of the *polis*. It was not to grant each his or her own voice. Tiresias did not demand to speak, or to be heard. He claimed the right to answer, which is to participate.

THE WILL TO BELIEVE

Postmodernism is too grand in its characterization of power, of which there are, in truth, many kinds. As Shalin (1993) articulates so well, there is power as oppression, domination, and control over others, the sort that postmodernism is concerned to overcome; but there is also power as empowerment and control of self, and this sort implies agency, individuation, and mastery of one's predicament. He argues that it is not a Nietzschean "will to power" that dri-

ves us, but a Jamesian "will to believe" that we can bring to the indeterminacy of the world in which we live some order, or sense, or
sanity; that we can find in it causes and consequences, reasons and
meanings; and that these can be communicated to others who are
interested to know of them.

Shucking authority is certainly relevant to adolescent risk involvement. Some teenagers, although not many, went so far as to
cast their parents as oppressors, and their risks as acts of liberation.
The language and metaphors of war and warfare are not unfamiliar
to children or parents when it comes to describing what takes place
between them on the battlefields of adolescence. Adolescents struggle for power, surely, but what they linger over and cling to is not
power for its own sake, but mastery of their own knowledge and circumstance: "So that *I* can know what I can do, instead of her always telling me"; "it proves something to yourself—that you can do
it"; "more and more it's a conscious effort at experience and
growth." They seem less intent on seizing power than declaring that
they are capable of holding the reins. What bubbles to the surface,
finally, is adolescents' will to believe that they can handle it.

A CONSPIRACY OF UNDERSTANDING

It is no surprise that Baldwin bows in William James's direction, toward his "will to believe," (James, 1897/1956), in the course of describing the experimental, forward reaching aspect of knowledge as
the belief that its speculations and hypotheses can become truths.
And although Baldwin's position on the social embeddedness of all
knowledge is settled and plain,[1] Crapanzano's (1979) work, perhaps
because it is more contemporary, conveys more explicitly the semiotic character of the process. He describes a "conspiracy of understanding" that people enter when they negotiate a shared reality.
People must believe that others will understand the reasons, meanings, and motives of what they do and say. They must believe that

---

[1]This is not to suggest that Baldwin is in any way dismissive of the social nature
of knowledge construction. He insists that all knowledge is public property,
never private possession, and that a person's knowledge is first and finally an
index of their social fitness.

others understand them as they understand themselves. This entails "casting the other to cast oneself" (p. 192), which is to cast oneself for the other and in the light of the other.

As partners in risk, adolescents enter a conspiracy of understanding of the most blatant sort. They show their commitment to one another, or try to get closer, or to stay close, or to know each other in a different way. They make memories and secrets to share and tell. They affirm who they are, and also who they are not. Risks are avatars of a liminal self—the self embodied—and on this account instrumental in acquiring self and other. As Peirce (1977) notes, "the signs of the self, its manifestations, *are* the real self, which emerges along with the external world by a process of fallible inference" (original italics).

Because the personal is cognate with the canonical, because, as Peirce writes, matter is "mind hidebound with habits," causality cannot be understood as a movement of some competence, norm, or value from a social to a personal plane. External information, accepted wisdom, good or bad manners, what it means to be a redneck or a preppie or a tree-hugger, these are not transported from outside to inside. Both of these "places" are personal and social. Thus, it makes no sense to speak of "peer pressure" as an external force that pushes a child into risky behavior (Lightfoot, 1992), or as something that can be deflected by just saying "no." And it is worrisome that some teenagers seem to have more insight into the complexities of the process than do the adults who would protect them from it. (Recall, in this context, the young man who notes that "the idea of peer pressure is a lot of bunk . . . everyone else would be doing it and you'd think, 'Hey . . . they seem to be having a good time—now why wouldn't I do this?' ") Likewise, it makes little sense to think that adolescents will be discouraged from taking particular risks simply because they have been exposed to information about the dangers involved. Interventions that aim to fix the kid (e.g., just say no) or fix the environment (e.g., just install condom dispensers in school washrooms) are shallow solutions that follow from dualistic conceptions of children and the contexts in which their actions have meaning.

All of this is to say that there is something inevitable in the fact that as the cabbage is changed into rabbit, it is the cabbage—not Mr. MacGregor's watering can—that beckons to be nibbled. Crapanzano's conspiracy of understanding, and other like-minded concepts, help to bury old dualisms in favor of something that recognizes the systemic, internal relations that hold between children and their webs of cultural truth, belief, value, and identification. Rather than a movement from outside to inside, the ongoing internalization and externalization that constitute mind and matter are better considered as a form of sociocognitive entrainment. To entrain, as I understand it, means to entangle. It means also, and more rarely, according to my *Webster's*, to "draw after oneself." This meaning permits a view of the child's reality as a complex interweaving of experience, a net, but it includes a provision for retaining the hand that casts it (Baldwin, 1908, p. 415).

We are dealing, first and finally, with the question of how to characterize the relationship between developing individuals and the changing cultural contexts in which they act. There would appear to be two general approaches in the social sciences (Lightfoot, in press-c). By one, the individual is considered to be part of a social whole, and development tends toward confluence, synchrony, analogy, and coregulation. That is, the interactional complexity of the whole is taken to be more than the sum of its constituent parts; more, that is, than the actions of individuals. Meaning, from this perspective, is manifested at the level of the group; it emerges as the actions of component individuals connect and become synchronized, rhythmic, and self-reproducing. Individual action, in and of itself, is inherently unintelligible, and is brought to heel within a field of interaction. The appeal of this approach lies in its willing submission to our desire to locate human action in cultural context: It focuses attention on process and dynamic, time and directionality, the relational movement toward stable meanings. The difficulty that undercuts it all, however, is that viewing the individual as part of a social whole disallows any talk of subjectivity, reflexivity, and critique, without which actions have direction, but they lack purpose; they have order and stability, but lack commitment; and they have dynamics, but lack drama.

Another approach is to construe the individual as an ensemble of social relations, and development as tending toward transformation, reconstruction, synthesis, and critique. This approach recaptures the subjectivity so often eclipsed by the cognitive atheism of contemporary social research. To view individuals ensembles of social relations is to place them at the center of their own action, and to care about the interpretive and constructive processes by which meanings are generated and become realities extending beyond the local contexts of their making. This has the effect of introducing a determinacy of meaning at the level of the individual act. Action *is* the composition of meaning, not just part of a larger process of meaning construction in which meaning is taken as an epiphenomenon to the action itself. A determinacy of meaning at the level of the act denies the congruence between signifier and signified, between that which is represented and the vehicle of representation. It denies that the letter compelleth the spirit (see also Hirsch, 1976).

Instead, meaningful action is taken as a mechanism of individual and sociocultural development, and this is because of its inherent duality and reflexivity. It organizes, frames, composes, comments on, and thereby transforms mere experience into a structure of experience. Thus, the difference between the two approaches—the individual as part of a social whole and the individual as an ensemble of social relations—really turns on the issue of reflexivity and the duality of action. To acknowledge the difference is to permit distinctions between mimicry and mime, identification and individuation, singularity and subjectivity, and these distinctions are important if our aim is to understand not only the reproduction of cultural and canonical forms, but their transformation into personal meanings.

Early in the book, I related the comment of a teenager who believed that adults' conceptions of peer pressure are "completely off," as are their lessons on how to resist it:

> "What I heard about peer pressure all the way through school is that someone is going to walk up to me and say, 'Here, drink this and you'll be cool.' It wasn't like that at all. . . . They have no idea what we're up against."

At that time, and in an effort to respond, I promised to try to give at least some sense of what they are "up against." In order to appreciate more fully what they are up against, we need to take stock of how adolescents wrap their acts in interpretations. Jessor and Jessor made the point many years ago (1975) that if we want teenagers to stop drinking alcohol, we should sever the symbolic connection between alcohol and maturity. We may question the practicality of his suggestion, but not the point of it. Risks are taken not for their own sake, but because they carry and communicate particular meanings. The "careless rapture" that accompanies play in all of its guises comes from shaping, forming, and composing material, and to give some account of playing and risk-taking on these terms is an interpretive task.

And what can such an epistemology offer to those of us concerned about the safety and well-being of children? I have argued here that risk-taking is natural and necessary to psychic life and development, but there is a double narrativity at work. On the one hand, risk-taking is but an example of the universal imaginative mode of interpretive activity; it is play, drama, cultural experience. On the other hand, however, risk-taking provides specific experiences that take form as shared narrative—as singular events or patterns of behavior that become icons of social identity—and it is here that we are inclined to believe that we might intervene. We ask, reasonably, why must the risk be drinking and driving, or tripping on acid, or having unprotected intercourse, or carrying a weapon? Why can't children pursue physical or intellectual challenge, or take risks that might be socially or politically redemptive? Some teenagers do. The logic of "functional equivalence" undergirds this reasoning, and also the recent popularity of adventure programs for delinquent youth. We would like to control or channel adolescents' behavior so that they may take risks, certain ones, without the danger of becoming injured, infected, drug addicted, pregnant, diseased, or censured from school or community. But we cannot provide children with opportunities for safe risk-taking. We can only provide them with opportunities for experience, realizing that out of these they will construct something remarkable that will become their lives.

References

Abrahams, R. (1986). Ordinary and extraordinary experience. In V. Turner & E. Bruner (Eds.), *The anthropology of experience*. Chicago: University of Illinois Press.

Addams, J. (1910). *The spirit of youth and the city streets*. New York: Macmillan.

Arnett, J. (1992). Reckless behavior in adolescence: A developmental perspective. *Developmental Review, 12*, 339–373.

Bakhtin, M. (1981). *The dialogic imagination* (M. Holquist, Ed.; C. Emerson, Trans.). Austin: University of Texas Press.

Bakhtin, M. (1986). *Speech genres and other late essays* (C. Emerson & M. Holquist, Eds.; V. W. McGee, Trans.). Austin: University of Texas Press.

Baldwin, J. M. (1906). *Thought and things: A study of the development and meaning of thought: Vol I. Functional logic*. New York: Macmillan.

Baldwin, J. M. (1908). *Thought and things: A study of the development and meaning of thought: Vol II. Experimental logic, or genetic theory of thought*. New York: Macmillan.

Baldwin, J. M. (1911). *Thought and things: A study of the development and meaning of thought: Vol III. Interest and art*. New York: Macmillan.

Bateson, G. (1972). *Steps to an ecology of mind*. New York: Ballantine Books.

Baumrind, D. (1987). A developmental perspective on adolescent risk taking in comtemporary America. In C. Irwin (Ed.), *Adolescent social behavior and health* (New Directions for Child Development, No. 37). San Francisco: Jossey-Bass.

Baumrind, D. (1989). Rearing competent children. In W. Damon (Ed.), *Child development today and tomorrow*. San Francisco: Jossey-Bass.

Bell, N., & Bell, R. (1993). Introduction. In N. Bell & R. Bell (Eds.), *Adolescent risk taking*. Newbury Park, CA: Sage.

Bentham, J. (1802/1931). *The theory of legislation*. London: Kegan Paul.

Bergson, H. (1911). *Creative evolution.* New York: Henry Holt.

Bretherton, I. (1989). Pretense: The form and function of make-believe play. *Developmental Review, 9,* 383–401.

Briggs, J. (1992). Mazes of meaning: How a child and a culture create each other. In W. Corsaro & P. Miller (Eds.), *Interpretive approaches to children's socialization* (New Directions for Child Development, No. 58). San Francisco: Jossey-Bass.

Britt, C., & Campbell, W. (1977). Assessing the linkage of norms, environments and deviance. *Social Forces, 56,* 532–550.

Bronner, S. (1988). *American children's folklore.* Little Rock, AR: August House.

Brown, B. (1990). Peer groups and peer cultures. In S. Feldman & G. Elliott (Eds.), *At the threshold: The developing adolescent.* Cambridge, MA: Harvard University Press.

Brown, B., Lohr, M. & Trujillo, C. (1990). Multiple crowds and multiple life styles: Adolescents' perceptions of peer-group stereotypes. In R. Muuss (Ed.), *Adolescent behavior and society: A book of readings.* New York: McGraw-Hill.

Bruner, J. (1986). *Actual minds, possible worlds.* Cambridge, MA: Harvard University Press.

Bruner, J. (1987). Life as narrative. *Social Research, 54,* 11–32.

Bruner, J. (1990). *Acts of meaning.* Cambridge, MA: Harvard University Press.

Buck-Morss, S. (1987). Piaget, Adorno and dialectical operations. In J. M. Broughton (Ed.), *Critical theories of psychological development.* New York: Plenum Press.

Burke, K. (1966). *Language as symbolic action: Essays on life, literature, and method.* Berkeley: University of California Press.

Cairns, R., Cairns, B., & Neckerman, H. (1989). Early school drop out: Configurations and determinants. *Child Development, 60,* 1437–1452.

Cairns, R., Cairns, B., Neckerman, H., Gest, S., & Gariépy, J. (1988). Social networks and aggressive behavior: Peer support or peer rejection? *Developmental Psychology, 24,* 815–823.

Cassirer, E. (1946). *The myth of the state.* New Haven, CT: Yale University Press.

Chandler, M. (1987). The Othello effect: Essay on the emergence and eclipse of skeptical doubt. *Human Development, 30,* 137–159.

Chandler, M. (1993). Contextualism and the post-modern condition: Learning from Las Vegas. In S. Hayes, L. Hayes, H. Reese, & T. Sarbin (Eds.), *Varieties of scientific contextualism.* Reno, NV: Context Press.

Chapman, M. (1991). The epistemic triangle. In M. Chandler & M. Chapman (Eds.), *Criteria for competence*. Hillsdale, NJ: Erlbaum.

Chaucer, G. (1963). *Canterbury tales* (V. Hopper, Trans.). New York: Barron's.

Cole, M. (1992). Context, modularity, and the cultural constitution of development. In L. T. Winegar & J. Valsiner (Eds.), *Children's development within social context: Vol. 2. Research and methodology*. Hillsdale, NJ: Erlbaum.

Connolly, J., & Keutner, T. (Eds.). (1988). *Hermeneutics versus science? Three German views*. Notre Dame, IN: University of Notre Dame Press.

Crapanzano, V. (1979). The self, the third, and desire. In B. Lee (Ed.), *Psychosocial theories of the self*. New York: Plenum Press.

Crites, S. (1986). Storytime: Recollecting the past and projecting the future. In T. Sarbin (Ed.), *Narrative psychology: The storied nature of human conduct*. New York: Praeger.

Cvetkovich, G., Grote, B., Bjorseth, A., & Sarkissian, J. (1975). On the psychology of adolescents' use of contraceptives. *Journal of Sex Research, 11*, 256–270.

Dembo, R., Schmeidler, J., & Burgos, W. (1979). Factors in the drug involvement of inner-city junior high school youth: A discriminant analysis. *International Journal of Social Psychology, 25*, 92–103.

Dewey, J. (1920/1957). *Reconstruction in philosophy*. Boston: Beacon Press.

Dewey, J. (1922). *Human nature and conduct*. New York: Henry Holt.

DiBlasio, F., (1986). Drinking adolescents on the roads. *Journal of Youth and Adolescence, 15*, 173–188.

Dilthey, W. (1900/1976). The development of hermeneutics. In H. Rickman (Ed.), *Dilthey: Selected writings*. Cambridge, England: Cambridge University Press.

Dunphy, C. (1963). The social structure of urban adolescent peer groups. *Sociometry, 26*, 230–246.

Elkind, D. (1978). Understanding the young adolescent. *Adolescence, 13*, 127–134.

Erikson, E. (1963). *Childhood and society*. New York: Norton.

Erikson, E. (1965). Youth: Fidelity and diversity. In E. Erikson (Ed.), *The challenge of youth*. New York: Anchor Books.

Erikson, E. (1968). *Identity: Youth and crisis*. New York: Norton.

Fein, G. (1989). Mind, meaning, and affect: Proposals for a theory of pretense. *Developmental Review, 9*, 345–363.

Fielding, H. (1749/1963). *Tom Jones*. New York: Washington Square Press.

Fine, G. A. (1992). The depths of deep play: The rhetoric and resources of morally controversial leisure. *Play and Culture, 5*, 246–251.

Fornäs, J. (1995). Youth, culture, and modernity. In J. Fornäs & G. Bolin (Eds.), *Youth culture in late modernity*. London: Sage.

Frost, J., & Wortham, S. (1988, July). The evolution of American playgrounds. *Young Children*, pp. 19–28.

Furby, L., & Beyth-Marom, R. (1992). Risk-taking in adolescence: A decision making perspective. *Developmental Review, 12*, 1–44.

Gadamer, H. (1975). *Truth and method.* New York: Seabury Press.

Gardner, W. (1993). A life-span rational-choice theory of risk taking. In N. Bell & R. Bell (Eds.), *Adolescent risk taking.* Newbury Park, CA: Sage.

Gariépy, J. (1995). The evolution of a developmental science: Early determinism, modern interactionism, and a new systemic approach. In *Annals of child development* (Vol. 11). London: Jessica Kingsley.

Garvey, C., & Kramer, T. (1989). The language of social pretend play. *Developmental Review, 9*, 364–382.

Gaskins, S., Miller, P., & Corsaro, W. (1992). Theoretical and methodological perspectives in the interpretive study of children. In W. Corsaro & P. Miller (Eds.), *Interpretive approaches to children's socialization.* (New Directions for Child Development, No. 58). San Francisco: Jossey-Bass.

Geertz, C. (1972). Deep play: Notes on the Balinese cockfight. *Daedalus, 101*, 1–27.

Geertz, C. (1973). *The interpretation of cultures.* New York: Basic Books.

Geertz, C. (1983). *Local knowledge.* New York: Basic Books.

Geertz, C. (1986). Making experiences, authoring selves. In V. Turner & E. Bruner (Eds.), *The anthropology of experience.* Chicago: University of Illinois Press.

Gergen, K. (1988). If persons are texts. In S. Messer, L. Sass, & R. Woolfolk (Eds.), *Hermeneutics and psychological theory: Interpretive persepctives on personality, psychotherapy, and psychopathology.* New Brunswick, NJ: Rutgers University Press.

Gergen, K., & Gergen, M. (1983). Narratives of the self. In T. Sarbin & K. Scheibe (Eds.), *Studies in social identity.* New York: Praeger.

Gillis, J. (1974). *Youth and history: Tradition and change in European age relations.* New York: Academic Press.

Giordano, P., Cernkovich, S., & Pugh, M. (1986). Friendships and delinquency. *American Journal of Sociology, 91*, 117–120.

Gould, S. (1987). *Time's arrow, time's cycle: Myth and metaphor in the discovery of geological time.* Cambridge, MA: Harvard University Press.

Gower, J. (1987). Introduction to ordination techniques. In P. Legendre & L. Legendre (Eds.), *Developments in numerical ecology* (NATO ASI Series, Vol. G14). Berlin: Springer-Verlag.

Grahame, P., & Jardine, D. (1990). Deviance, resistance, and play: A study in the communicative organization of trouble in class. *Curriculum Inquiry, 20*, 283–304.

Green, J. (1989). Analyzing individual differences in development: Correlations and cluster analysis. In J. Colombo & J. Fagan (Eds.), *Individual differences in infancy*. Hillsdale, NJ: Erlbaum.

Habermas, J. (1979). *Communication and the evolution of society*. Boston: Beacon Press.

Habermas, J. (1988). *On the logic of the social sciences*. Cambridge, MA: MIT Press.

Hall, G. S. (1904). *Adolescence: Its psychology and its relations to physiology, anthropology, sociology, sex, crime, religion, and education*. New York: Appleton-Century-Crofts.

Hallowell, A. (1955). The self and its behavioral environment. In *Culture and experience*. Philadelphia: University of Pennsylvania Press.

Hankiss, A. (1981). Ontologies of the self: On the mythological rearranging of one's life-history. In D. Bertauz (Ed.), *Biography and society: The life history approach in the social sciences*. Newbury Park, CA: Sage.

Harré, R. (1975). Images of the world and societal icons. In K. Knorr, H. Strasser, & H. Zilian (Eds.), *Determinants and controls of scientific thought*. Dordrecht, The Netherlands: Reidel.

Harré, R. (1991). What is real in psychology: A plea for persons. *Theory and Psychology, 2*, 153–158.

Harré, R., & Madden, E. (1975). *Causal powers*. Totowa, NJ: Littlefield Adams.

Harré, R., & van Langenhove, L. (1991). Varieties of positioning. *Journal for the Theory of Social Behavior, 21*, 393–407.

Hartup, W. (1983). Peer relations. In P. Mussen (Ed.), *Handbook of child psychology: Vol. IV. Socialization, personality, and social development*. New York: Wiley.

Heidegger, M. (1927/1976). *Being and time*. New York: Harper & Row.

Hesse, H. (1925/1968). *Demian*. New York: Bantam.

Hirsch, E. (1976). *The aims of interpretation*. Chicago: University of Chicago Press.

Holland, D. (1991) How cultural models become desire: A case study of American romance. In R. D'Andrade & C. Strauss (Eds.), *Human motives and cultural models*. Cambridge, England: Cambridge University Press.

Holland, D. & Valsiner, J. (1988). Cognition, symbols, and Vygotsky's developmental psychology. *Ethos, 16*, 247–272.

Howard, A. (1985). Ethnopsychology and the prospects for a cultural psychology. In G. White & J. Kirkpatrick (Eds.), *Person, self and experience: Exploring Pacific ethnopsychologies*. Berkeley: University of California Press.

Hubba, G., Wingard, J., & Bentler, P. (1979). Beginning adolescent drug

use and peer and adult interaction patterns. *Journal of Consulting and Clinical Psychology, 47,* 265–276.

Huizinga, J. (1938/1955). *Homo Ludens.* Boston: Beacon Press.

Inhelder, B., & Piaget, J. (1958). *The growth of logical thinking from childhood to adolescence.* New York: Basic Books.

Irwin, C. (Ed.). (1987). *Adolescent social behavior and health* (New Directions for Child Development, No. 37). San Francisco: Jossey-Bass.

Irwin, C. (1990). The theoretical concept of at-risk adolescents. *Adolescent Medicine, 1,* 1–14.

Irwin, C. (1993). Adolescence and risk taking: How are they related? In N. Bell & R. Bell (Eds.), *Adolescent risk taking.* Newbury Park, CA: Sage.

Irwin, C., & Millstein, S. (1987). The meaning of alcohol use in early adolescents. *Pediatric Research, 21,* 175–187.

James, W. (1897/1956). *The will to believe.* New York: Dover.

Jessor, R. (1987). Risky driving and adolescent problem behavior: An extension of problem-behavior theory. *Alcohol, Drugs, and Driving, 3,* 1–11.

Jessor, R. (1992). Risk behavior in adolescence: A psychosocial framework for understanding and action. *Developmental Review, 12,* 374–390.

Jessor, R., Chase, J., & Donovan, J. (1980). Psycho-social correlates of marijuana use and problem drinking in a national sample of adolescents. *American Journal of Public Health, 70,* 604–613.

Jessor, R., & Jessor, S. (1975). Adolescent development and the onset of drinking. *Journal of Studies on Alcohol, 36,* 27–51.

Kandel, D. (1978). Homophily, selection, and socialization in adolescent friendships. *American Journal of Sociology, 84,* 427–436.

Kandel, D., & Lesser, G. (1972). *Youth in two worlds.* San Francisco: Jossey-Bass.

Kegeles, S., Millstein, S., & Adler, N. (1987). The transition to sexual activity and its relationship to other risk behaviors. *Journal of Adolescent Health Care, 8,* 303.

Kerney, R. (1988). Ricoeur and the hermeneutic imagination. In T. Kemp & D. Rasmussen (Eds.), *The narrative path: The later works of Paul Ricoeur.* Cambridge, MA: MIT Press.

Kett, J. (1977). *Rites of passage.* New York: Basic Books.

Kiell, N. (1959). *The adolescent through fiction: A psychological approach.* New York: International Universities Press.

Klintzer, M., Rossiter, C., Gruenewald, P., & Balinsky, M. (1987). Determinants of youth attitudes and skills towards which drinking/driving prevention programs should be directed (Report to the National Highway Traffic Safety Administration, Contract No. DTNH 22–84–C-07248). *Status Report, 16,* 1–11.

Koch, S. (1981). The nature and limits of psychological knowledge: Lessons of a century qua "science." *American Psychologist, 36,* 257–269.

Kupersmidt, J., & Patterson, C. (1991). Childhood peer rejections, aggression, withdrawal, and perceived competence as predictors of self-reported behvior problems in preadolescence. *Journal of Abnormal Child Psychology, 19,* 427–449.

Ladd, G. (1983). Social networks of popular, average, and rejected children in school settings. *Merrill–Palmer Quarterly, 29,* 283–307.

Lastovicka, J., Murry, J., Joachimstahler, E., Bhalla, G., & Scheurich, J. (1987). A lifestyle typology to model young male drinking and driving. *Journal of Consumer Research, 14,* 157–263.

Lee, B., & Hickmann, M. (1983). Language, thought, and self in Vygotsky's developmental theory. In B. Lee & G. Noam (Eds.), *Developmental approaches to the self.* New York: Plenum Press.

Legendre, P. (1976). An appropriate space for clustering selected groups of Western North American *Salmo. Systematic Zoology, 25,* 193–195.

Lemann, N. (1989, November). Stressed out in suburbia. *Atlantic Monthly,* pp. 34–48.

Leontiev, A. (1971). Preface. In L. Vygotsky, *The psychology of art.* Cambridge, MA: MIT Press.

Levitt, M., & Selman, R. (1996). The personal meaning of risk behavior: A developmental pespective on friendship and fighting in early adolescence. In G. Noam & K. Fischer (Eds.), *Development and vulnerability in close relationships.* Mahwah, NJ: Erlbaum.

Lewin, K. (1933). Environmental forces. In C. Murchison (Ed.), *Handbook of child psychology.* Worcester, MA: Clark University Press.

Lightfoot, C. (1992). Constructing self and peer culture: A narrative perspective on adolescent risk taking: In L. Winegar & J. Valsiner (Eds.), *Children's development within social context: Vol 2. Research and methodology.* Hillsdale, NJ: Erlbaum.

Lightfoot, C. (in press-a). The clarity of perspective: Adolescent risk-taking, fantasy, and the internalization of cultural identity. In B. Cox & C. Lightfoot (Eds.), *Sociogenetic perspectives on internalization.* Mahwah, NJ: Erlbaum.

Lightfoot, C. (in press-b). Slouching towards Paradigm Land: A review of *Youth culture in late modernity. Culture and Psychology.*

Lightfoot, C. (in press-c). Transforming the canonical cowboy: Notes on the determinacy and indeterminacy of children's play and cultural development. In A. Fogel, M. Lyra, & J. Valsiner (Eds.), *Dynamics and indeterminism in developmental and social processes.* Hillsdale, NJ: Erlbaum.

Lightfoot, C., & Folds-Bennett. T. (1992). Description and explanation in developmental research: Separate agendas. In J. Asendorph & J. Valsiner (Eds.), *Stability and change in development: A study of methodological reasoning.* Newbury Park, CA: Sage.

Lightfoot, C., & Valsiner, J. (1992). Parental belief systems under the influence: Social guidance of the construction of personal cultures. In I. Sigel, A. McGillicuddy-DeLisi & J. Goodnow (Eds.), *Parental belief systems: The psychological consequences for children* (2nd ed.). Hillsdale, NJ: Erlbaum.

Lipps, T. (1903). *Aesthetik.* Hamburg: Voss.

Lopes, L. (1987). Between hope and fear: The psychology of risk. In L. Berkowitz (Ed.), *Advances in experimental social psychology* (Vol. 20). New York: Academic Press.

Lopes, L. (1993). Reasons and resources: The human side of risk taking. In N. Bell & R. Bell (Eds.), *Adolescent risk taking.* Newbury Park, CA: Sage.

Lorenz, K. (1972). In M. Piers (Ed.), *Play and development: A symposium with contributions by Jean Piaget, Peter H. Wolff, Ren Spitz, Konrad Lorenz, Lois Barclay Murphy, Erik Erikson.* New York: Norton.

Lyng, S. (1993). Dysfunctional risk taking: Criminal behavior as edgework. In N. Bell & R. Bell (Eds.), *Adolescent risk taking.* Newbury Park, CA: Sage.

Lyotard, J. (1984). *The postmodern condition: A report on knowledge.* Minneapolis: University of Minnesota Press.

May, R. (1991). *The cry for myth.* New York: Norton.

McCord, J. (1990). Problem behaviors. In S. Feldman & G. Elliott (Eds.), *At the threshold: The developing adolescent.* Cambridge, MA: Harvard University Press.

McDermott, J. (Ed.). (1967) . *The writings of William James: A comprehensive edition.* New York: Random House.

McKnight, A., Preusser, D., Psotka, J., Katz, D., & Edwards, J. (1979). *Youth alcohol safety education criteria development.* Alexandria, VA: National Public Services Research Institute.

Mead, G. (1934). *Mind, self, and society.* Chicago: University of Chicago Press.

Millstein, J. S., & Irwin, C. (1987). Accident-related behaviors in adolescents: A biopsychosocial view. *Alcohol, Drugs, and Driving, 4,* 21–29.

Minick, N. (1987). The development of Vygotsky's thought: An introduction. In R. Rieber & A. Carton (Eds.), *The collected works of L. S. Vygotsky: Vol. 1. Problems of general psychology.* New York: Plenum Press.

Moreno, J. (1934). *Who shall survive: A new approach to the problem of human in-*

terrelations. Washington DC: Nervous and Mental Disease Publishing Co.

Nicolopoulou, A. (1993). Play, cognitive development, and the social world: Piaget, Vygotsky, and beyond. *Human Development, 36*, 1–23.

Opie, I., & Opie, P. (1959). *The lore and language of school children.* Oxford, England: Oxford University Press.

Ortega y Gasset, J. (1914/1961). *Meditations on Quixote.* New York: Norton.

Overton, W. (1991). The structure of developmental theory. In H. Reese (Ed.), *Advances in child development and behavior.* New York: Academic Press.

Overton, W. (1994). The arrow of time and the cycle of time: Concepts of change, cognition, and embodiment. *Psychological Inquiry, 5,* 215–237.

Peacock, J., & Holland, D. (1993). The narrated self: Life stories in process. *Ethos, 21,* 367–383.

Peirce, C. (1977). Semiotics and significs. In C. S. Hardwick (Ed.), *The correspondence between Charles S. Peirce and Victoria Lady Welby.* Bloomington: Indiana University Press.

Piaget, J. (1955). *The language and thought of the child.* New York: Meridian Books.

Piaget, J. (1962). *Play, dreams and imitation in childhood.* New York: Norton.

Piaget, J. (1965/1995). *Sociological studies.* New York: Routledge.

Piaget, J. (1972). *The child and reality.* New York: Grossman.

Renninger, K. A., & Winegar, L. T. (1985). Emergent organization in expert–novice relationships. *Genetic Epistemologist, 14,* 14–20.

Ricoeur, P. (1972). The model of the text: Meaningful action considered as text. Social Research, 38, 529–562.

Ricoeur, P. (1976). *Interpretation theory: Discourse and the surplus of meaning.* Fort Worth: Texas Christian University Press.

Ricoeur, P. (1983). Can fictional narratives be true? In A. T. Tymieniecka (Ed.), *Analecta Husserliana* (Vol. 14). Dordrecht, The Netherlands: Reidel.

Rieber, R., & Carton, A. (Eds.). (1987). *The collected works of L. S. Vygotsky: Vol. 1. Problems of general psychology.* New York: Plenum Press.

Rogoff, B. (1990). *Apprenticeship in thinking: Cognitive development in social context.* New York: Oxford University Press.

Rommetveit, R. (1991) Axiomatic features of a dialogic approach. In I. Markova & K. Foppa (Eds.), *The dynamics of dialogue.* New York: Springer-Verlag.

Rorty, A. (1976). *The identities of persons.* Berkeley: University of California Press.

Rosaldo, R. (1986). Ilongot hunting as story and experience. In V. Turner & E. Bruner (Eds.), *The anthropology of experience*. Chicago: University of Illinois Press.

Rousseau, J. (1762/1911). *Emile* (B. Foxly , Trans.). London: Dent.

Rubin, K., Fein, G., & Vandenberg, B. (1983). Play. In P. Mussen (Ed.), *Handbook of child psychology: Vol. IV. Socialization, personality, and social development*. New York: Wiley.

Sandars, N. K. (Trans.). (1960). *The epic of Gilgamesh*. Baltimore: Penguin Books.

Sarbin, T. (1986). The narrative as a root metaphor for psychology. In T. Sarbin (Ed.), *Narrative psychology: The storied nature of human conduct*. New York: Praeger.

Sarbin, T. (1990). Metaphors of unwanted conduct: A historical sketch. In D. Leary (Ed.), *Metaphors in the history of psychology*. Cambridge, England: Cambridge University Press.

Scheibe, K. (1986). Self-narrative and adventure. In T. Sarbin (Ed.), *Narrative psychology*. New York: Praeger.

Schlegel, A., & Barry, H. (1991). *Adolescence: An anthropological inquiry*. New York: Free Press.

Schwartzman, H. (1978). *Transformations: The anthropology of children's play*. New York: Plenum Press.

Secord, P. (1986). Explanations in the social sciences and in life situations. In D. Fiske & R. Shweder (Eds.), *Metatheory in social science: Pluralisms and subjectivities*. Chicago: University of Chicago Press.

Selman, R. (1980). *The growth of intepersonal understanding*. New York: Academic Press.

Shalin, D. (1993). Modernity, postmodernism, and pragmatist inquiry: An introduction. *Symbolic Interaction, 16*, 303–332.

Shedler, J., & Block, J. (1990). Adolescent drug use and psychological health: A longitudinal inquiry. *American Psychologist, 45*, 612–630.

Sherif, M., Harvey, O., White, B., Hood, W., & Sherif, C. (1961). *Inter-group conflict and cooperation: The Robbers Cave experiment*. Norman: University of Oklahoma Press.

Sherif, M., & Sherif, C. (1964). *Reference groups*. New York: Harper & Row.

Shibutani, T. (1955). Reference groups as perspectives. *American Journal of Sociology, 60*, 562–569.

Silbereisen, R., & Eyferth, K. (1986). Development as action in context. In R. Silbereisen, K. Eyferth, & G. Rudinger (Eds.), *Development as action in context: Problem behavior and normal youth development*. New York: Springer-Verlag.

Silbereisen, R., Eyferth, K. & Rudinger, G. (Eds.). (1986). *Development as ac-

tion in context: Problem behavior and normal youth development. New York: Springer-Verlag.

Sneath, P. & Sokal, R. (1973). *Numerical axonomy: The principles and practice of numerical classification.* San Francisco: Freeman.

Stacey, T., & Davies, T. (1970). Drinking behavior in childhood and adolescence: An evaluative review. *British Journal of Addictions, 65,* 203–212.

Sutton-Smith, B. (1966). Piaget on play: A critique. *Psychological Review, 73,* 104–110.

Sutton-Smith, B. (1981). *A history of children's play.* Philadelphia: University of Pennsylvania Press.

Sutton-Smith, B. (1984). Text and context in imaginative play and the social sciences. In F. Kessel & A. Goncu (Eds.), *Analyzing children's play dialogues* (New Directions for Child Development, No. 25). San Francisco: Jossey-Bass.

Sutton -Smith, B., & Kelly-Byrne, D. (1984). The idealization of play. In P. Smith (Ed.), *Play in animals and humans.* London: Basil Blackwell.

Taylor, C. (1985). *Human agency and language: Philosophical papers 1.* New York: Cambridge University Press.

Titchener, E. (1910). *Textbook of psychology.* New York: Macmillan.

Trilling, L. (1971). *Sincerity and authenticity.* Cambridge, MA: Harvard University Press.

Trommsdorff, G. (1986). Future time oreintation and its relevance for development as action. In R. Silbereisen, K. Eyferth, & G. Rudinger (Eds.), *Development as action in context.* New York: Springer-Verlag.

Turner, V. (1982). *From ritual to theatre: The human seriousness of play.* New York: Wiley.

Turner, V. (1986). Dewey, Dilthey, and drama: An essay in the anthropology of experience. In V. Turner & E. Bruner (Eds.), *The anthropology of experience.* Chicago: University of Illinois Press.

Valsiner, J. (1987). *Culture and the development of children's actions: A cultural-historical theory of developmental psychology.* New York: Wiley.

Valsiner, J. (1988). *Developmental psychology in the Soviet Union.* Sussex, England: Harvester Press.

Valsiner, J. (1989). *Human development and culture: The social nature of personality and its study.* Lexington, MA: Lexington Books.

Valsiner, J. (1991). Construction of the mental: From the cognitive revolution to the study of development. *Theory and Psychology, 1,* 477–494.

Valsiner, J. (1992). Making of the future: Temporality and the constructive nature of human development: In G. Turkewitz & D. Devenney (Eds.), *Time and timing in development.* Hillsdale, NJ: Erlbaum.

Valsiner, J. (1994a). Co-constructivism: What is (and is not) in a name? In P. van Geert & L. Mos (Eds.), *Annals of theoretical psychology* (Vol. 10). New York: Plenum Press.

Valsiner, J. (1994b). Reflexivity in context: Narratives, hero-myths, and the making of histories in psychology. In A. Rosa & J. Valsiner (Eds.), *Historical and theoretical discourse in social–cultural studies.* Madrid: Fundación Infancia y Aprendizaje.

Valsiner, J. (1994c). Irreversibility of time and the construction of historical developmental psychology. *Mind, Culture, and Activity, 1,* 25–42.

Valsiner, J., & Cairns, R. (1992). Theoretical perspectives on conflict and development. In C. Shantz & W. Hartup (Eds.), *Conflict in child and adolescent development.* Cambridge, England: Cambridge University Press.

Valsiner, J., & van der Veer, R. (1988). On the social nature of human cognition: An analysis of the shared intellectual roots of George Herbert Mead and Lev Vygotsky. *Journal for the Theory of Social Behavior, 18,* 117–136.

Valsiner, J., & van der Veer, R. (1993). The encoding of distance: The concept of the Zone of Proximal Development and its interpretations. In R. Cocking & K. Renninger (Eds.), *The development and meaning of psychological distance.* Hillsdale, NJ: Erlbaum.

van der Veer, R., & Valsiner, J. (Eds.). (1994). *The Vygotsky reader.* Cambridge, MA: Blackwell.

Violato, C., & Wiley, A. (1990). Images of adolescence in English literature: The middle ages to the modern period. *Adolescence, 25,* 253–264.

Vygotsky, L. (1971). *The psychology of art.* Cambridge, MA: MIT Press.

Vygotsky, L. (1977). Play and its role in the mental development of the child. In M. Cole (Ed.), *Soviet developmental psychology: An anthology.* White Plains, NY: Sharpe.

Vygotsky, L. (1979). The genesis of higher mental functions. In J. Wertsch (Ed.), *The concept of activity in Soviet psychology.* Armonk, NY: Sharpe.

Vygotsky, L. (1987). *The collected works of L. S. Vygotsky: Vol. 1. Problems of general psychology* (R. Rieber & A. Carton, Eds.). New York: Plenum Press.

Vygotsky, L. (1994). Imagination and creativity of the adolescent. In R. van der Veer & J. Valsiner (Eds.), *The Vygotsky reader.* Cambridge, MA: Blackwell.

Watson-Gegeo, K. (1992). Thick explanation in the ethnographic study of child socialization: A longitudinal study of the problem of school for Kwara'ae (Solomon Islands) Children. In W. Corsaro & P. Miller (Eds.), *Interpretive approaches to children's socialization* (New Directions for Child Development, No. 58). San Francisco: Jossey-Bass.

Werner, H., & Kaplan, B. (1984). *Symbol formation*. Hillsdale: NJ: Erlbaum.

Wertsch, J. (1985). *Vygotsky and the social formation of mind*. Cambridge, MA: Harvard University Press.

Wertsch, J. (1991). Dialogue and dialogism in a socio-cultural apporach to mind. In I. Markova & K. Foppa (Eds.), *The dynamics of dialogue*. New York: Springer-Verlag.

Wertsch, J. (1993). Commentary. *Human Development, 36*, 168–171.

Wertsch, J., & Minick, N. (1990). Negotiating sense in the zone of proximal development. In M. Schweel, C. Maher, & N. Fagley (Eds.), *Promoting cognitive growth over the life span*. Hillsdale, NJ: Erlbaum.

Willis, P. (1977). *Learning to labour*. London: Saxon House.

Winegar, L. T. (in press). Can "internalization" be more than a magical phrase?: Notes toward the contstructive negotiation of this process. In B. Cox & C. Lightfoot (Eds.), *Sociogenetic perspectives on internalization*. Mahwah, NJ: Erlbaum.

Winegar, L. T., Renninger, K. A., & Valsiner, J. (1989). Dependent-independence in adult–child relationships. In D. A. Kramer & M. J. Bopp (Eds.), *Transformation in clinical and developmental psychology*. New York: Springer-Verlag.

Winnicott, D. (1971). *Playing and reality*. New York: Tavistock.

Wolfenstein, M. (1953). Trends in infant care. *American Journal of Orthopsychiatry, 23*, 120–130.

Wolfenstein, M. (1955). The fun morality. In M. Mead & M. Wolfenstein (Eds.), *Childhood in contemporary cultures*. Chicago: University of Chicago Press.

Youniss, J., & Smollar, J. (1985). *Adolescent relations with mothers, fathers, and friends*. Chicago: University of Chicago Press.

Zigler, E., Taussig, C., & Black, K. (1992). Early childhood intervention: A promising preventative for juvenile delinquency. *American Psychologist, 47*, 997–1006.

Author Index

Abrahams, R., 57, 167n.
Addams, J., 18, 167n.
Adler, N., 22, 172n.
Arnett, J., 24, 25, 34, 167n.

B

Bakhtin, M., 56, 59–65, 69, 112, 167n.
Baldwin, J. M., 42, 53, 54, 65, 68, 91–93, 157, 158, 164, 167n.
Balinsky, M., 22, 26, 172n.
Barry, H., 15, 176n.
Bateson, G., 69, 79, 167n.
Baumrind, D., 20, 21, 167n.
Bell, N., 22, 167n.
Bell, R., 22, 167n.
Bentham, J., 84, 167n.
Bentler, P., 27, 140, 171n., 172n.
Bergson, H., 65, 168n.
Beyth-Marom, R., 23, 25, 170n.
Bhalla, G., 29, 173n.
Bjorseth, A., 25, 169n.
Black, K., 21, 179n.
Block, J., 21, 176n.
Bretherton, I., 87, 168n.
Briggs, J., 49, 168n.
Britt, C., 27, 168n.
Bronner, S., 77, 78, 168n.
Brown, B., 27, 134, 140, 168n.
Bruner, J., 2, 12, 41, 48, 56, 168n.
Buck-Morss, S., 87, 88, 168n.

Burgos, W., 27, 169n.
Burke, K., 43, 69, 90, 132, 168n.

C

Cairns, B., 27, 139, 140, 168n.
Cairns, R., 27, 52, 139, 140, 168n., 178n.
Campbell, W., 27, 168n.
Carton, A., 40, 175n.
Cassirer, E., 76, 168n.
Cernkovich, S., 26, 170n.
Chandler, M., 159, 168n.
Chapman, M., 155, 169n.
Chase, J., 26, 172n.
Chaucer, G., 16, 169n.
Cole, M., 51, 169n.
Connolly, J., 39, 169n.
Corsaro, W., 35, 170n.
Crapanzano, V., 162, 169n.
Crites, S., 2, 57, 169n.
Cvetkovich, G., 25, 169n.

D

Davies, T., 28, 105, 177n.
Dembo, R., 27, 169n.
Dewey, J., 18, 74, 169n.
DiBlasio, F., 22, 26, 169n.
Dilthey, W., 24, 38, 169n.
Donovan, J., 26, 172n.
Dunphy, C., 30, 134, 140, 169n.

Subject Index

Adolescent egocentrism, 34, 35
Adventure
    age of, 63
    and experience, 58
    gender differences in preference
        for, 125
    quest for, 18
    time, 61, 63, 65
Aesthetics
    and experience, 2, 54, 159
    and play, 70, 84
Autonomy, 11, 20, 56, 59, 114

B

Behaviorism, 44, 49
Bildungsroman, 12, 60, 64

C

Causality, 21, 24, 45, 46, 71, 153,
    156, 163
Cluster sampling, 3, 139
Cognitivism, 44, 45, 49
Contextualism, 159
Cultural development, 25

D

Decision-making, 23, 29
Deep play, 67, 83–85
    risk-taking as, 84, 98, 125
    see also Play

Deep time, 65, 66
Dependent-independence, 114
Depression, 105
Discourse, authoritative and
    internally persuasive, 112,
    113
Drama, 8, 12, 49, 53, 57, 164
Dramatic engagement, 129
Drug and alcohol use, 23, 27–29,
    33, 99–103, 109, 115,
    125–127
DWI, 25, 26

E

Edgework, 58
Empiricism, 24, 35, 47, 60
Experience
    cultural, 12, 96, 156, 166
    depth of, 56, 59, 66
    dramatic, 57
    etymology of, 57
    structured, 2, 48, 165
    risk-taking as, 2, 58, 97–99,
    108
    transformative, 55, 56
    and transitional phenomena, 91
    meaning of, 35, 52, 56, 61

F

Fantasy, 9, 55, 95, 118
Folklore, 76–79